AF898271

MINDFULNESS FOR PSYCHOSIS

Mindfulness for Psychosis

A GROUP THERAPY APPROACH

Paul Chadwick
Katherine Newman-Taylor
Nicola Abba

Foreword by Jon Kabat-Zinn

THE GUILFORD PRESS
New York London

Copyright © 2027 The Guilford Press
A Division of Guilford Publications, Inc.
www.guilford.com

All rights reserved

Except as noted, no part of this book may be reproduced, translated, stored in a retrieval system, or transmitted, in any form or by any means, electronic, mechanical, photocopying, microfilming, recording, or otherwise, without written permission from the publisher.

Printed in the United States of America

This book is printed on acid-free paper.

For product and safety concerns within the EU, please contact *GPSR@taylorandfrancis.com*, Taylor & Francis Verlag GmbH, Kaufingerstraße 24, 80331 München, Germany.

Last digit is print number: 9 8 7 6 5 4 3 2 1

LIMITED DUPLICATION LICENSE

These materials are intended for use only by qualified mental health professionals.

The publisher grants to individual purchasers of this book nonassignable permission to reproduce all materials for which photocopying permission is specifically granted in a footnote. This license is limited to you, the individual purchaser, for personal use or use with clients. This license does not grant the right to reproduce these materials for resale, redistribution, electronic display, or any other purposes (including but not limited to books, pamphlets, articles, video or audio recordings, blogs, file-sharing sites, internet or intranet sites, and handouts or slides for lectures, workshops, or webinars, whether or not a fee is charged). Permission to reproduce these materials for these and any other purposes must be obtained in writing from the Permissions Department of Guilford Publications.

This publication is intended to provide helpful and informative material. It is not intended to diagnose, treat, cure, or prevent any health problem or condition, nor is it intended to replace the advice of a health professional. No action should be taken based solely on the contents of this book. Always consult your physician or qualified health care professional on any matters regarding your health and before adopting any suggestions in this book or drawing inferences from it.

The authors and publisher specifically disclaim all responsibility for any liability, loss, or risk, personal or otherwise, which is incurred as a consequence, directly or indirectly, from the use or application of any contents of this book.

Any and all product names referenced within this book are the trademarks of their respective owners. Always read all information provided by the manufacturers' product labels before using their products. The authors and publisher are not responsible for claims made by manufacturers.

Library of Congress Cataloging-in-Publication Data is available from the publisher.

ISBN 978-1-4625-6450-7 (paperback) ISBN 978-1-4625-6451-4 (cloth)

We are deeply grateful to the many people
with distressing psychosis who have trusted us,
taught us about living with psychosis, and learned
mindfulness alongside us. This book is dedicated
to them all in gratitude and with a hope that
this guidance empowers other clinicians to support more
people with psychosis to find greater self-acceptance,
calm, and connection, and to be themselves more fully
wherever their personal recovery takes them.

About the Authors

Paul Chadwick, PhD, is Professor of Clinical Psychology at the University of Bath, United Kingdom. Since the 1990s, his pioneering research has advanced psychological understanding and therapy of distressing psychosis, including showing how delusions are amenable to psychological therapy, establishing the foundational concept of the omnipotence of voices, and developing mindfulness for psychosis. Dr. Chadwick is a recipient of the M. B. Shapiro Lifetime Achievement Award, the Award for Distinguished Contributions to Professional Psychology, and the May Davidson Award from the British Psychological Society.

Katherine Newman-Taylor, PhD, is Professor of Clinical Psychology and Cognitive Behavior Therapy at the University of Southampton, United Kingdom, and Consultant Clinical Psychologist in the National Health Service. Her clinical and research interests are in working with people with psychosis. Dr. Newman-Taylor draws on attachment, mindfulness, and recovery principles to strengthen cognitive-behavioral approaches to living well with voices, paranoia, and other unusual experiences.

Nicola Abba, PhD, is Deputy Director of the Cognitive Behavior Therapy Training Programs at the University of Southampton, United Kingdom, and Consultant Clinical Psychologist in the National Health

Service. During her doctoral research, Dr. Abba developed the first psychological theory of how people learn to respond mindfully to distressing psychosis experiences. Her clinical practice since the early 2000s has focused on both mindfulness and cognitive-behavioral approaches to working with people with psychosis and other severe and enduring mental health problems, particularly in acute inpatient settings.

Foreword

We have no idea how what we call "the mind" creates a world "out there" in which we can navigate for the most part effortlessly, and an interior world as well, accompanied by a sense that there is a me, a self, who is having experiences. It is a colossal mystery (Pollan, *A World Appears*). Moreover, those inner and outer worlds are highly ordered, curated as they are to a very large degree via our senses, of which there are more than five (Kabat-Zinn, *Coming to Our Senses*). Animals also have interior lives, often spoken of as the mystery of "what it is like to be . . ." an elephant, a rhinoceros, a bat, a dog or a cat (Pollan, *A World Appears*; Yong, *An Immense World*), or maybe even a paramecium or other single-celled creature.

In the domain of us humans, mostly it goes well. Remarkably well in fact. Everything works relatively seamlessly, and we go about our complex lives with a remarkable degree of inner and outer homeostatic integration, along with a sense of freedom, well-being, and undisputed agency. We fit in more or less, we belong more or less, and that belonging usually unfolds within a larger circle of family, friends, colleagues, strangers, language, culture, the natural world. We don't give it a thought.

What is more, our particular human brand of sentience is pretty seamless. We call it normal, even though we are normally hardly aware of our interior thought worlds, our emotions, and the sense of having a body, of proprioception and interoception. We have interior and exterior lives that seamlessly integrate experience across all these domains, allowing us to be "normal," to function effectively as a human being within a family, a complex society, and a larger world.

Indeed, when it comes to training in mindfulness, a foundational feature of the work described in this book, beginning meditators are often astonished by the realization that, as human beings, we all have voices in our heads that drive us to one degree or another. They are called thoughts. As soon as we take up the regular practice of meditation, the first thing we discover, almost immediately, is just that: that the mind has a life of its own. It wanders. It streams. It cascades . . . an endless waterfall of thoughts and emotions, memories and fantasies. It could be the voice of a parent that we hear speaking to us out of the past, or of a good friend. Sometimes the thoughts are creative and insightful, sometimes seriously problematic, even destructive. More often than not, they are mundane in the extreme, just endless laundry lists of what we should be doing, or wish we had done. Sometimes they are freighted with unhelpful emotions. Meditation teachers call this *the cascading mind.*

And if this discovery is made in a class with other people, as in mindfulness-based stress reduction (MBSR) or mindfulness-based cognitive therapy (MBCT), or in the program described in this volume, we soon learn that this is in fact the case for everybody. That makes it "normal," if not always optimal. You set yourself the task of, say, simply attending to the flow of your breathing, just feeling it wherever the sensations are most vivid for you, perhaps at the nostrils or in the expanding and receding of the abdomen, and lo and behold, almost immediately your mind wanders. And what does it wander into? Thinking. Narratives. Memories. Images. Imaginings. Sometimes pleasant, sometimes seriously unpleasant, sometimes neither, just blah, in one way or another, it can all be subsumed under the rubric of "the story of me."

It turns out it is non-trivial to sustain one's attention, no matter who you are, for even the duration of one inbreath and one outbreath, never mind over an extended stretch of time. It bears repeating that this mental activity is absolutely normal. In fact, it defines "normal." Virtually everybody's mind functions in this way, usually with absolutely no awareness of it. The meditative traditions sometimes refer to it as "the untrained mind."

This is where the cultivation of mindfulness, or moment-to-moment *non-judgmental* awareness, can play a powerful role in establishing some degree of perspective, emotional balance, and a healthy sense of agency. It is also where compassion comes in. We can be kind to ourselves because things are just as they are. It is not our fault. Liberative insights and some compassion for oneself can arise as a result of realizing this and coming to terms with the actuality of it.

The work described in this book is firmly grounded in the cultivation of mindfulness/heartfulness as a formal meditation practice and a way of being. Its singular, boundary-stretching aim is to provide it as a training program for people diagnosed with psychosis. It is a brave foray into the possibility of coming to terms with things as they are in one's life and in one's mind, starting from where one finds oneself in the present moment, even when the challenges being faced are, on their face, staggering. For a diagnosis of psychosis is in many ways congruent with other major mental health challenges, such as major depressive illness, for instance, itself a disorder of thinking that has been shown by Segal, Williams, and Teasdale (*Mindfulness-Based Cognitive Therapy for Depression*) to be amenable to healing through MBCT. What these psychiatric diagnoses have in common is the often cruel, self-destructive, deluded, yet seemingly compelling and self-reinforcing interior narratives the mind tends to fabricate that endlessly taunt and demean the bearer.

Psychosis can be described as a symptom or condition rather than a single diagnosis. It refers to a loss of contact with consensus reality. It can include hallucinations (e.g., hearing voices), delusions (strongly held false beliefs), as well as disorganized thinking or speech. It can manifest under many different circumstances—in brief stress reactions, or with severe depression, bipolar disorder, substance use, certain medical or neurological illnesses, and more.

In the brave work described here in the exquisite detail required of a treatment manual, the authors make the case that mindfulness can be an effective therapeutic approach in and of itself in healing psychosis, and map out in great detail for interested clinicians how to go about it. Healing, of course, does not imply *curing*, but rather, *a coming to terms* with things as they are, and optimizing one's ongoing well-being and ability to cope with challenges to whatever degree possible. In other words, learning to live and live well within the challenges such a condition presents.

While it may be challenging in the extreme, what people with this diagnosis are carrying (the root meaning of the word "to suffer") is workable in exactly the way the authors describe. The evidence and high-resolution clinical guidance they offer clearly demonstrate that when an appropriate, sensitive, and welcoming framework and holding environment is created, mindfulness as both a formal meditation practice and as a moment-by-moment way of being in the world can be of profound value in the lives of people with this diagnosis coming to terms with the various challenges, inner and outer, that they face, often on a moment-by-moment basis. It provides clinicians interested in doing this kind of work all the support and guidance they might require—in parallel, of course, with the requirement of having their own ongoing mindfulness practice, an absolutely essential and foundational element of this treatment approach.

When people are referred to MBSR with a broad range of medical diagnoses, as a rule we tend not to look at the diagnosis at first, but instead, to apprehend the human being who is showing up, and how they respond to the open-ended question: What brings you here today? This invites deep listening and full presence on the part of the clinician right off the bat, and a welcoming and friendly willingness to encounter the person in their fullness. In other words, it not only invites but also *requires* the full presence of the clinician in their own humanity, rather than solely in their authoritative role. After all, mindfulness means being fully present in open awareness, that is, embodied and open-hearted. The word itself conjures *heartfulness*, reflected in the fact that in many Asian languages, the words for mind and heart are the same.

As in MBSR and MBCT, in this work the distinction between reacting mindlessly versus responding mindfully in the moment to any event arising in one's mind or in the world plays a central role and is demonstrated to be hugely liberating for people plagued by thoughts, impulses, and habitual tendencies that will simply not go away. Learning the *how* of living with these unwanted visitors and not be overwhelmed by them is by no means easy. It is an unfolding process grounded in a willingness to bravely *turn toward* and face what one most wants to squash or escape from or surrender to, and in the process, discover new degrees of freedom in living one's life without succumbing to one's condition. Here, the authors make the important point right up front that they are not describing a mindfulness-based *therapy*. Rather mindfulness itself, as a practice and as a way of life, *is* the therapy.

Their process, manualized here in great detail, allows the practitioner new to this work to introduce the practice of mindfulness as an effective and potentially transformative way of being for people suffering from psychosis. However, as is the case for MBSR and MBCT, and all other therapeutic approaches that are based on the cultivation of mindfulness through actual *practice*, it is essential for the therapist to have their own robust and ongoing mindfulness practice and work to deepen it through study, learning from more experienced mindfulness teachers, and periodically attending teacher-led meditation retreats.

May this book provide guidance for all health professionals hoping to be optimally effective in helping people with the diagnosis of psychosis to recognize their humanity, their belonging, and their capacity to navigate the twists and turns of their inner and outer lives with skill, consistency, and compassion for themselves.

JON KABAT-ZINN, PhD
Northampton, Massachusetts

REFERENCES

Pollan, M. (2026). *A world appears: A journey into consciousness.* Penguin Press.

Kabat-Zinn, J. (2005). *Coming to our senses: Healing ourselves and the world through mindfulness.* Hachette Books.

Yong, E. (2022). *An immense world: How animal senses reveal the hidden dimensions around us.* Penguin Random House.

Segal, Z. V., Williams, J. M. G, & Teasdale, J. D. (2013). *Mindfulness-based cognitive therapy for depression* (2nd ed.). Guilford Press.

Preface

We three began working together in 2001 and it was over the next decade that we developed mindfulness for psychosis. Together we facilitated the first mindfulness for psychosis groups and published the qualitative and quantitative research that established the theoretical and practical underpinnings of mindfulness for psychosis. It was a creative, inspiring, and deeply rewarding time for us. Collaborating closely again to write this book has been just as creative, inspiring, and rewarding. Throughout, we have been blessed to collaborate with many, many generous and talented people who have shaped the theory and practice of mindfulness for psychosis presented here, and we are grateful to them all.

As we disseminated our work and raised awareness of the potential for mindfulness to ease the tyranny of psychosis, many people asked if we had a manual to support them for running these groups. We had written about aspects of mindfulness for psychosis—the two-circles model, the core process of change, the importance of metacognitive insight, and group factors. We had also written about how mindfulness can be integrated within a broader person-based cognitive therapy for psychosis (Chadwick, 2006) and cognitive-behavioral therapy for psychosis (Newman-Taylor & Abba, 2015, 2018). However, nowhere had we presented guidance on how to facilitate mindfulness for psychosis groups in sufficient depth to convey the theoretical and practical underpinnings in full, and in sufficient detail to equip and empower people to facilitate these groups.

We began working on this book in 2021. At first it was slow going, but we stuck to it! When Senior Editor Jim Nageotte reached out from The Guilford Press, we realized that the time was right: We had a publisher who cared about people with psychosis, valued this work, and wanted to support us to disseminate this approach. We are grateful to Jim, Developmental Editor Jane Keislar, and all at The Guilford Press, for their trust, impetus, and expert editorial guidance. We also thank David Araci for his enthusiasm and thoughtful comments on an earlier draft. Finally, we would like to express our heartfelt gratitude to Jon Kabat-Zinn, both for his generosity in writing the foreword, which contextualizes the book so well, and for making our work possible.

At times this has been a challenging book to write. The elements of mindfulness for psychosis are so deeply interconnected that it can be hard to describe any one aspect without diverting into potentially unhelpful discussion of others. Processes such as stepping back, choice, and acceptance, and group factors such as universality and being oneself more fully, are inseparable facets of one whole, one gestalt. It has been quite a balancing act, seeking to articulate the various elements of mindfulness, and describe the intrinsic links among them, without getting lost in the myriad connections that confuse rather than clarify guidance for people learning to deliver these groups. We have done our best with this tightrope walk.

We have tried always to keep in mind two things when writing this book. The first is the question *What will be most helpful to people learning to facilitate mindfulness for psychosis groups?* You, our reader, have accompanied us as we grappled with this, and we hope this guide proves useful to you. Second, we have held close to our hearts the people with psychosis we have worked with over many years. Meeting them as people and learning mindfulness together have been some of the most rewarding moments of our careers, and we have sought to do our best by them.

This book does not describe a mindfulness-based therapy. Here, mindfulness *is* the therapy. This is different from describing how mindfulness practice may be integrated within, say, cognitive-behavioral therapy or another psychological therapy. While we hope the book supports and enriches the practice of people facilitating mindfulness-based therapies for psychosis, the approach presented here stands alone. Furthermore, this is a *group* therapy. In our work and in this book, we have focused on and embraced the therapeutic benefits of being part of a group when learning mindfulness, and in particular the experience of a common humanity that can arise in these groups, and can transform our lives as a result.

A note on practicalities: we have recorded variations of the core mindfulness practice to support you as you learn to deliver the groups. These audio recordings are available at *www.guilford.com/chadwick-materials* and we explain how to make the best use of these recordings in Chapter 8. Regarding terminology, in most of this book, we use "he" or "she" when discussing specific individuals, aligned with their gender. The names used are anonymized and represent the range of people we have worked with. If we discuss an individual without giving a name, we have used "they" or "their."

Contents

I. THE CONTEXT AND THEORY OF MINDFULNESS FOR PSYCHOSIS

II. MINDFULNESS IN PRACTICE

III. MINDFULNESS FOR PSYCHOSIS GROUPS: THE 8-WEEK PROGRAM

IV. SUPPORTING ONGOING RECOVERY AND DEVELOPING AS FACILITATORS

Purchasers of this book can download and print copies of select materials, as well as stream and download audio files, at *www.guilford.com/chadwick-materials* for personal use or use with clients (see copyright page for details).

I

The Context and Theory of Mindfulness for Psychosis

1

The Tyranny of Psychosis

"I always thought I heard voices because I was a nasty, horrible person, just not a human being, not worthy of not having voices. I was lost in a different world, scared and fighting voices all the time, just trying to survive. But with the help of the group, I've come to accept that I have voices, that it's no good fighting them all the time. I feel in control more, more confident, and have started setting myself goals. Now when I go out, I'm aware of where I am and the people around me—it feels good. I realize now that there is good in everybody, that hearing voices doesn't make us awful people, we are the same as everybody else."—SANDRA

The impact of psychosis on the person and their family and friends is profound and far-reaching. Indeed, it is hard to overstate the degree to which many people feel overwhelmed and tyrannized by their psychosis. People describe being tormented by experiences such as voices and paranoia, defeated by self-criticism and low self-esteem, and undone in losing a coherent sense of themselves. This can leave people feeling powerless, traumatized, utterly alone, and scarcely able to cope. For some, the impact of psychosis, often compounded by trauma and stigmatized societal reactions, can lead people to feel less than human. This is the challenge that inspired the development of mindfulness for psychosis: Might mindfulness be a means of supporting people to find some peace and freedom from the distress, tyranny, and dehumanization of psychosis?

Schizophrenia and Psychosis

Perhaps more than any other mental health diagnosis, *schizophrenia*, or *psychosis*, can seem terrifying, devastating. Clinically and culturally, since first recorded accounts, schizophrenia and psychosis have been conceived as beyond comprehension (Woods, 2011). Jaspers (1913/1997) described schizophrenia as lying on the other side of the *abyss* that separates what can from what cannot be understood. More recently, Lacan (1993) assumed that psychosis lacks coherent meaning, leading nowhere: "At the heart of the psychoses there is a dead end" (p. 184). In many societies, schizophrenia is arguably the most feared and stigmatized of all mental health diagnoses.

It is hard for us not to internalize and fear this *otherness* of psychosis, this pervasive sense of incomprehensibility. It is therefore understandable when mental health professionals and mindfulness facilitators who are considering working therapeutically with people with psychosis feel some apprehension and self-doubt. These reactions arise for most of us at times, and we do not need to judge or avoid acknowledging them. As you read this book, if anxiety or self-doubt should arise, try to hold these lightly. Simply by opening this book, you are expressing your curiosity about this work and compassion for people with psychosis, and this is a wonderful place to start.

The Tyranny of Psychosis: Omnipotent, Malevolent Voices

While not everyone finds psychosis experiences distressing, people coming to mental health services and mindfulness for psychosis groups typically come with highly distressing and disturbing voices (*auditory hallucinations*), thoughts (*delusions*), or images (*visual hallucinations*).

Lee heard three powerful, evil voices, all male. The voices were almost constant and always seemed to be nearby, talking about him to one another. Sometimes the voices would trigger traumatic memories from his past. The voices threatened to harm him and his parents and sisters, and used foul language to refer to deeply distressing past events. Lee was in a state of intense fear most of the time and convinced this was happening only to him. The threats to harm his family caused a great deal of fear and fueled his paranoia. Lee had lost his job and separated from his partner. He spent much time alone and felt isolated and depressed. There was no one he believed he could talk to about what was happening. The voices were not people he knew or recognized. Lee was not religious but thought the voices must be some kind of evil spirit. He believed he was being punished but was too frightened to make sense of why they were tormenting him—he was frozen with fear much of the time. Lee often ran up and down the stairs in the tower block where he lived, trying to escape the voices. On a few occasions he tried to confront them, knocking on the doors of neighboring flats where he thought the voices might be hiding. Once, he fled London and ended up in an unfamiliar town many miles from home. He briefly thought he was free of the voices but described how they had followed him a day or so later. Lee was sure they would kill him one day soon.

While some voices can be benevolent, most of the people we work with hear voices that are experienced as extremely powerful or omnipotent and malevolent (Chadwick & Birchwood, 1994). Voices are usually experienced as *not me* and as coming from other people or beings—the typically tyrannical relationship with voices is inherently interpersonal. Some people recognize their voices as people from their lives, past or present, whereas for others the voice's identity is unknown. People often attribute a God like or supernatural quality to voices and perceive malevolent voices to be a type of evil spirit or devil.

Voices may comment on what the person is currently doing or thinking, and often seem to know all about them (Chadwick & Birchwood, 1994). They commonly allude, or even refer directly, to people's most private, shameful, and traumatic experiences, and memories, thoughts, and fears, leading the person to believe that the voices can read their mind. This apparent *omniscience* leaves people feeling exposed and vulnerable, and erodes a sense of having a private self. Voices' omnipotence is often reinforced by upsetting or fantastic images over which the person also believes they have little or no control. This gives voices an apparent *superhuman* quality and leaves people feeling powerless and overwhelmed (Chadwick & Birchwood, 1994). As Martin said, "*They've got a hold over you, these voices. They will make you very angry, they will make you distressed, angry, you can even start crying. It won't let you go, it just won't let you lie there and rest, they're always at you. They're at you 24 hours of the bloody day.*"

Many people feel that voices rule their lives. Many resist and fight back, or seek to somehow appease their voices, but these coping strategies are exhausting and do not work well. If there is any respite, voices usually return and once again overwhelm the person, leaving them feeling trapped and helpless, with no means of escape. People experience themselves not only as having no control over the voices but as having lost control and agency over their own lives. When offering mindfulness for psychosis groups, it is crucial that we keep in mind the common felt sense of voice omnipotence, omniscience, and malevolence, and to recognize that most people experience their voices as being qualitatively different from the distressing thoughts, images, feelings, and other unpleasant sensations that we all have.

The Tyranny of Psychosis: Paranoia and Persecution

Paul was tormented by a sense of persecution, not voices. He believed he was the victim of a vast conspiracy involving thousands of people. This paranoid belief (or *persecutory delusion*) had become all consuming. He rarely left home, and when he did, it seemed to him that every person he saw was part of the conspiracy and was giving him a personal, coded message through their choice of clothing or body language. On returning home, he would spend hours recalling people he had seen, their clothes and mannerisms, searching for clues as to what they had been communicating.

Paul would notice unusual physical sensations in his body and believed these were caused by his persecutors using some kind of satellite to observe him, test his body, and read his mind. He was convinced that this "*emotional and psychological torture*" was damaging his brain and body. There were days when all he could do was hide away for hours on end and "think and think and think"—trying to figure out what was being done to him and why. Although this unhelpful repetitive thinking was exhausting and frustrating, he persisted, clinging to a hope that if he could work out what was behind it all, perhaps he could somehow put a stop to the persecution.

Paul had dropped out of college around the time his paranoia emerged and had not worked nor studied since. He had lost contact with his few friends, and stopped meeting his mother and sister, who he thought must know what was being done to him even though they denied this. He felt a near constant sense of threat and exposure. He trusted no one; mistrust and suspiciousness had become his default mode. Paul felt powerless, trapped, and more than anything, frightened. At times he became suicidal, no longer able to bear the persecution and desperate to bring it to an end.

The Tyranny of Psychosis: Images and Other Experiences

It is important to recognize the impact of psychosis experiences other than voices and paranoia. Images are common and often linked to and reinforce a voice's power and omniscience. Kaitlin found the many images that intruded into her awareness to be even more distressing and more difficult to live with than the omnipotent, malevolent voices she heard threatening and criticizing her, and commanding her to harm or kill herself.

Distressing voices, images, and beliefs, particularly paranoia, are among the most widely recognized and characteristic experiences, or *symptoms*, of psychosis. These are certainly among the most common psychosis experiences reported by people attending our mindfulness groups, though people may also experience grandiosity, confusion, and impoverished thinking, feeling, and motivation. For many, the voices, images, and paranoia are linked—for example, centering around a powerful, malevolent other—as was the case for Joseph: "*These experiences, they're kind of persecutory . . . I'll hear and sometimes see them, the three evil men. They torment me and sort of deride me. They destroyed my life, I was in and out of psychiatric wards, I was in hospital three times in one year. Some of the darkest moments of my life.*" Additionally, most people joining mindfulness groups also describe distressing non-psychosis experience, such as loss, depression, intrusive thoughts, trauma memories, and anxiety.

The Impact of Psychosis

For the people we see in mindfulness groups, psychosis impacts every aspect of their lives through frequent moments of debilitating fear, struggle, and despair. Many people like Lee live lives heavy with trauma and loss *before* the onset of psychosis, which then becomes another ongoing source of trauma that affects all areas of their life.

As the experiences of Lee and Paul illustrate, *devastating losses* often lie at the heart of psychosis (McCarthy-Jones et al., 2011). These include the loss of consensual reality, a coherent and acceptable sense of self, personal agency, physical security, and relationships with family and friends. Even individuals' inner worlds no longer seem private.

People with psychosis commonly perceive themselves to be viewed as less than human by others: their voices, perceived persecutors, past bullies and abusers, and society as a whole. Mental health care services can exacerbate these effects, whether through forced hospital admissions, medication, or denial of autonomy and choice (*epistemic injustice*; Larkin & Hutton, 2017). Health care staff and mindfulness facilitators can also internalize societal prejudice, fear, and dehumanizing attitudes toward people with psychosis. This process occurs even in relationships with family and friends:

> *"Once I told my best friend about the voices and images I get. She told me that I was mad, that no such things existed, and stopped being my friend. It really broke me. I had no one else that I could talk to. It made me feel the things I see and hear are not something a normal person would experience. I locked myself away from people, gave up work and study, lost my life. I felt like I don't have what it takes to be part of things that normal people do and like I shouldn't be existing."*—JOHN

The most profound loss effected by psychosis may be the perceived loss of common humanity. Psychosis, trauma, stigma, and isolation can result in people losing a sense of being a person at all and coming to view themselves as *less than* or *no longer human* (*self-dehumanization*; O'Brien-Venus et al., 2023)—that is, to place themselves on the far side of the abyss, separate from and unconnected to all others (Jaspers, 1913/1997):

> *"The thing is how the psychosis completely destroyed my sense of self, you know, my self-esteem, or my self-confidence. I lost my sense of self-respect and my sense of dignity and my sense of having human rights."*—JAY

In summary, people with psychosis experience devastating losses, often over many years, and can finally come to experience themselves as less than human. These effects are felt not only by the person with psychosis but by their families and friends. At times, professionals and others seeking to help can also feel at a loss when faced with the full impact of psychosis on all aspects of a person's life and self.

Might Mindfulness Bring Some Freedom from the Tyranny of Psychosis?

The answer to this lies in the nature of suffering and freedom from suffering. Some 2,500 years ago, the Buddha observed that suffering (distress) comes from a particular attitude and way of reacting to present-moment experience. Similarly, over 2,000 years ago, the Greek Stoic philosopher Epictetus reasoned that *people are disturbed not by the things that happen to them but by how they make sense of and react to what is happening.* In 20th-century Europe, Viktor Frankl arrived at the same conclusion while living under unimaginable tyranny in concentration camps—that the last of the *human freedoms* is to choose how to react in any situation.

The first contemporary secular mindfulness-based intervention, mindfulness-based stress reduction (MBSR; Kabat-Zinn, 1990), is based on this key observation. Working initially with people with severe and chronic pain, Kabat-Zinn explained that extremes of suffering were not inevitable consequences of physical sensations of pain in the body, but reflected a particular way of relating to pain, driven by non-acceptance, resistance, avoidance, and fear. This groundbreaking approach to Western mental health care showed that it is possible through mindfulness training for people to be free of suffering and despair, even when the physical sensations of pain remain.

It is important to recognize that to be mindful is not to stop responding emotionally to life; it is not to become cut off, unfeeling, or robotic. By letting go of reactive habits—such as avoidance, repetitive thinking, and resistance—we experience our lives *more fully*, and this includes moments of pain and sorrow, as well as moments of joy and connection.

While emotional and physical pain are part of human experience, we can learn to free ourselves from the additional burden of extremes of distress and suffering. Cognitive-behavioral therapy (CBT) and many other psychotherapies are built on exactly this premise (e.g., Beck et al., 1964, 1979): that while we do not get to choose all that happens to us in our lives, we can learn to choose how we respond. Life events and sensory experiences can bring pain and loss, but it is our enduring beliefs, attitudes, and reactions to our experiences that generate sustained extremes of distress and suffering, such as major depression and persistent anxiety. Segal, Williams, et al. (2002) developed mindfulness-based cognitive therapy (MBCT) initially for recurrent depression, by combining the principles of MBSR and CBT, demonstrating that it is possible to reduce relapse by learning to respond mindfully to transient low mood and streams of self-critical or hopeless appraisals that commonly arise.

CBT for psychosis is based on this same understanding of the origins of extreme distress and disturbance (Chadwick et al., 1996; Garety et al., 2001; Kingdon & Turkington, 2022; Morrison, 2001; Nelson, 2005). For example, an early cognitive model of voices showed that linked distress was predicted by *beliefs* about voices (that they were omnipotent, malevolent, and controlling) and *resistance* (e.g., efforts at distraction and avoidance, or fighting with them), indicating that reevaluation of beliefs and alternative reactions to voices could reduce distress (Chadwick & Birchwood, 1994). How people react to psychosis experience makes all the difference.

Mindfulness for psychosis stems from this same premise about the nature of suffering. This approach does not aim to *get rid* of voices, images, paranoid thoughts, and other psychosis experiences. Instead, we seek to foster alternative responses that ease distress, reconnect people with family and friends, and regain a sense of common humanity. There is now compelling evidence from both qualitative and quantitative studies that learning to relate mindfully to psychosis can ease distress and suffering (Abba et al., 2008; Ellett, 2024; Hodann-Caudevilla et al., 2020; Jansen et al., 2020; Liu et al., 2021; McGlanaghy et al., 2021).

Mindfulness for psychosis offers people a way to reduce distress and overwhelm, nurture self-acceptance and self-efficacy, and feel empowered to take steps toward personal recovery—that is, to free themselves from the tyranny of psychosis. In mindfulness for psychosis groups, change is based on trust and acceptance of people as fundamentally human and of intrinsic value.

2

Relating Mindfully to Psychosis

THE TWO-CIRCLES MODEL

The beginnings of this approach were prompted by considering whether mindfulness might enable people to change how they relate to psychosis experiences. Our intention was to develop a mindfulness intervention specifically for people with psychosis that would allow them to respond mindfully, moment by moment, to unpleasant voices, images, thoughts, and other experiences, and ascertain whether this reduced people's distress and facilitated self-acceptance. In short, could mindfulness enable people to free themselves from the tyranny of psychosis?

The 8-week mindfulness program has two linked theoretical foundations: the *two-circles model* (presented in this chapter), and the *core process of change* (see Chapter 3). The two-circles model describes and contrasts two ways of relating to an unpleasant psychosis experience—*distressing habitual reaction* and *mindful responding* (Chadwick, 2006; Chadwick et al., 2005). The core process of change describes the psychological process of moving from distressing reactivity to mindful responding (Abba et al., 2008).

The Two-Circles Model

Any application of mindfulness to specific disorders should be theoretically driven (Teasdale et al., 2003). Mindfulness is based on the premise that distress and suffering are not inherent aspects of certain (e.g., psychosis) events but mediated by how we react or respond to these events. Distress is alleviated by letting go of habitual self-defeating reactions and "paying attention in a particular way: on purpose, in the present moment and non-judgmentally" (Kabat-Zinn, 1994, p. 4). In mindfulness for psychosis, the intention is to be aware of psychosis experiences as they arise, just as they are, without reacting in ways that drive distress.

The development of mindfulness for psychosis was grounded in a clear conceptual framework: the two-circles model (see Figure 2.1). This describes how people relate *in the moment* to unpleasant psychosis (and non-psychosis) experiences or *sensations*. The model maps and contrasts defining attributes of habitual reaction and mindful responses to psychosis experiences.

Reaction describes relating to unpleasant experience in an immediate, automatic, habitual way—of being on *autopilot* (Segal, Williams, et al., 2002) or *thinking fast* (Kahneman, 2011), with little sense of control, personal agency, or decision making. By contrast, *response* describes the process of stepping back, seeing clearly what is present, and choosing how to relate to experiences as they arise. In this way, the two-circles model depicts how—in any moment that a person becomes aware of an unpleasant voice, image, thought, feeling, or other sensation—there is a

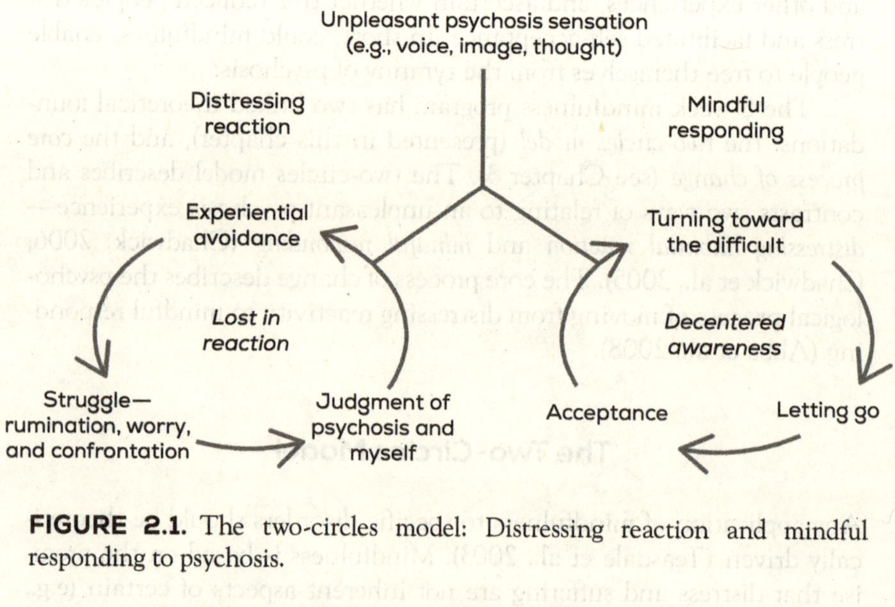

FIGURE 2.1. The two-circles model: Distressing reaction and mindful responding to psychosis.

potential choice. This choice is at the heart of mindfulness for psychosis: whether to lose oneself in distressing, exhausting, habitual reaction, or to observe the sensation, allow this to come into awareness, and then let it pass or fade without reacting. This choice is almost always outside people's awareness and understanding at the start of mindfulness groups, and the process of moving from distressing reactivity to mindful responding, the hard work involved in learning to step back and choose to respond differently, is discussed in the next chapter.

Sensations

The two-circles model describes processes that begin with awareness of an unpleasant sensation—perhaps an unpleasant voice, image, thought, feeling, or felt sense, for example, of being watched. In psychiatric classification systems, these experiences are viewed as *symptoms*. From a mindfulness perceptive, it can be helpful instead to view these as *sensations*. We have found that this immediately removes some of the difference or otherness associated with psychosis, and lays the foundation for extending mindfulness to other unpleasant experiences such as low mood and anxiety.

Sensations share certain attributes. They (1) belong to the person, (2) are tied to a particular site in the body, (3) are modality specific, and (4) occur in the present (Humphrey, 1993). While voices (*auditory hallucinations*) are most commonly reported by people who attend mindfulness groups, many are also distressed by images (*visual hallucinations*), sensations on the skin (*tactile hallucinations*), and smells and tastes (*olfactory/gustatory hallucinations*). It is important to note that psychosis experiences, such as voices, images, thoughts, and so on, are problems for the individual only if associated with distress or disturbance (Chadwick et al., 1996). When psychosis is causing distress or risk not to the person but to others around them, a different approach is likely needed.

The criterion of sensations *belonging to the person* might seem at odds with the experience of a voice, image, and thought as quintessentially *not me*. However, there is no inconsistency if we define a sensation as belonging to a person insofar as *this is happening to me*. For example, if I hear a phone ring, I do not assume I generated or wanted the sound, but recognize that the sensation of hearing ringing *belongs to me* (Chadwick, 2006).

While psychosis sensations *occur in the present*, most people are distressed even when voices are silent, images are absent, and persecutors seem to have abated. People with psychosis describe many moments of fear, dread, and defeat; anticipating the return of powerful, malevolent voices, images, or persecutors; worrying about where they are, what they are doing, and when they will return; or recalling and ruminating over what the voices and others have said, done, and meant. These unpleasant sensations of fear, dread, despair, and rumination can trigger the same distressing reactions as the psychosis experiences. For example, a person might worry about going out later in the day, knowing that their paranoia will escalate when preparing to leave the comparative safety of home. In this way, the impact of psychosis can be ever present, threatening and with no possibility of rest or escape.

A final feature of sensations, which comes from mindfulness traditions, is that they carry a *feeling tone* (*vedanā*). This is not the same as distress, which is laden with meaning and psychological reaction. A feeling tone is described simply as being pleasant (e.g., *apricity*—the warmth of sun on the skin on a cold day), unpleasant (e.g., physical pain), or neither pleasant nor unpleasant (neutral). In mindfulness groups, we do not deny or seek to change the feeling tone—a derogatory voice that is screaming abuse is likely to remain an unpleasant experience however a person learns to respond.

Avoidance

Experiential avoidance is a transdiagnostic reaction that occurs when a person is unwilling to remain in contact with sensations (Hayes, 1994). In relation to psychosis, experiential avoidance occurs in two main ways. First, when an unpleasant sensation is present, a person tries to take their attention away from it. This might involve ignoring or actively using a distraction method such as self-harm or listening to very loud music to drown out the voices. Second, many people with psychosis seek to prevent an unpleasant sensation entering awareness in the first place. For example, a person whose paranoia or agitated grandiosity is triggered by being around strangers might avoid leaving their home, and someone who sees malevolent images at night might use excessive alcohol, drugs, or sleep to block conscious awareness at these times. Avoidance is a key part of how people seek to resist omnipotent, malevolent voices, powerful persecutors, and other psychosis sensations.

Judging Sensations and the Self

Distress is also driven by judgments, particularly of unpleasant sensations and the self. It is important to remember that in psychosis an unpleasant voice, image, or other sensation is often experienced as another person or being—this *not-me* quality is a core part of the phenomenological experience of hallucinations and some forms of confusion (e.g., *thought insertion*). This means that for people with psychosis, judging an unpleasant sensation is often experienced as judging another person or being who has intruded into their mind.

Judgment of the self has two key qualities that we need to keep in mind when working with people with psychosis. First, it is typically "*all of me*," the entire self, that is judged as bad, flawed, worthless, a failure, and so on—that is, the judgment is global. Second, these judgments of the self seem (in the moment) to be fixed, or stable—the person believes this is "*just who I am*" and cannot be any different. Understandably, these global and stable judgments drive despair and hopelessness, as they seem to leave no room for change. The global and stable quality of self-judgments are often implicit and need to be drawn out during the guided discussion, or *inquiry*, that follows mindfulness practices. Self-critical judgments are often reinforced by experiences such as malevolent voices and memories of past trauma. Explicitly naming these judgments paves the way for self-acceptance—for example, that "*I am so much more than these voices, these memories.*"

Since beliefs about the self and others develop alongside each other, it is unsurprising, though important to keep in mind, that judgments of sensations and judgments of the self are typically connected. For example, when Usha gave her baby a bath, she would hear voices shouting, "*drown it, drown it, drown it.*" She was horrified by these words and voices (i.e., judging the sensations) and herself for being a terrible person, thinking, "*What kind of mother has this in her head?*" (i.e., judging herself).

Struggle: Rumination, Worry, and Confrontation

As we saw for Lee and Paul in Chapter 1, rumination, worry, and confrontation also drive distressing reactions to unpleasant psychosis experience. When people are not avoiding these sensations, they are often ruminating about their meaning and worrying about future consequences, exacerbating the distress. As Paul said of his paranoia: "*You just want to work it out, so you won't let go until you have.*" Distress can lead to angry confrontation with voices, images, and perceived persecutors. It is vital that we recognize that these reactions typically occur in the context of fear and overwhelm.

Being Caught and Lost in Reacting

Distressing reactions, depicted on the left-hand side of the two-circles model, is a dynamic process resulting in a distressed state of mind (cf. Williams, 2008). Avoidance, judgment, and struggle do not occur in a neat, linear process but arise in a disorderly way; the person's experience is of "*Distressfully leaping about in the space, reacting, reacting*" (Martin). These habitual reactions feed into one another, creating a vicious cycle that can quickly spiral: "*I lose my temper sometimes about something. That can happen. Your emotions go the other way, you start drawing them all in, you get that sort of whirlpool effect, which drags you down*" (Richard) and "*After 20 minutes, you're going to be screaming, breaking windows, throwing your shoes against the wall, banging your fists against the wall*" (Martin).

The person is caught—and lost—in this reactive process, without clear awareness of what is happening. Sandra, who heard multiple voices talking to one another about her and her life, vividly described this quality of being caught and lost in psychosis: "*The voices are there all the time and you're talking back to them but trying not to show it. So many times I've missed my stop on the underground [subway]. I'm in another world—completely unaware of where I am, who's around me, or anything.*"

The two-circles model helps bring a sense of order and understanding to what is typically experienced as being swept up in the chaos of uncontrolled reaction. Sharing the model helps to contain overwhelming feelings and support people to begin to recognize when they are caught up in reaction, the impact of this, and, crucially, any moments when they are not lost in familiar reactivity.

Well-worn habitual reactions come at considerable psychological costs in the short and long term. These reactions increase the intensity of psychosis experience—for example, voices become louder and more aggressive when voice hearers react with anger and confrontation (Romme & Escher, 1989), or become entangled in avoidance, rumination, and worry (e.g., Austin et al., 2015; Newman-Taylor et al., 2008;

Sellers et al., 2017). Images and persecutors can become more menacing when people try to push them out of mind, and relying on avoidance is associated with low mood and anxiety (Chadwick & Birchwood, 1994), and relapse (Gumley et al., 2008; Romme et al., 1992).

Having drawn out common habitual reactions, it is important to validate and normalize this way of relating to psychosis. The two-circles model is in no way saying that it was either a conscious choice or a mistake to react in the ways depicted on the left-hand side of the diagram. These are universal and automatic reactions to unpleasant and threatening experience. We are all hardwired to react in these ways; flight, fight, and freeze reactions evolved because they are adaptive when faced with immediate external threats—for example, an aggressive dog or being assaulted. However, when it comes to threatening or otherwise disturbing *internal* experiences, where escape is not possible, these reactions exacerbate rather than ameliorate distress and suffering (Williams, 2010).

Responding Mindfully to Unpleasant Psychosis Sensations: Decentered Awareness

In direct contrast to habitual reaction, responding mindfully is to step back and observe sensations (adopting a *decentered* perspective or awareness; Teasdale, 1993), allowing these to come into conscious awareness and then pass or fade without reacting or identifying with them (i.e., judging the self). Where reacting involves automatic, typically habitual action, responding involves a deliberate choice to turn toward that which is aversive. Each aspect of a mindful response to unpleasant psychosis sensations is in contrast to the corresponding elements of distressing reaction.

Rather than being caught and lost in distressing reaction, at the heart of mindful responding is a clear and grounded awareness of unpleasant psychosis sensations—that is, a moment in which the person is anchored in an awareness of the sensations arising. Before practicing mindfulness, Sandra would miss her underground [subway] stop, lost "*in another world*" of voices, paranoia, and confusion. After attending the group, she described a change: "*I'm much better now—I don't miss my stop. The voices are still there but I know where I am, I see the people around me, I get off when I need to.*"

The transdiagnostic concept of *decentering* is to be grounded in an awareness of the breath, body, or sensations (Segal, Teasdale, et al., 2002), "a process through which one is able to step outside of one's immediate experience, thereby changing the very nature of that experience" (Safran & Segal, 1996, p. 117). With practice people learn "rather than simply being their emotions, or identifying personally with negative thoughts and feelings [they can] relate to negative experiences as mental events in a wider context or field of awareness" (Teasdale et al., 2002, p. 276).

We have seen this process emerge in mindfulness groups. As Alison put it: "*Step back from your thoughts and feelings, become more aware of them*" and Steve: "*To me my normal state of affairs is I'm moving all the time, I'm running away or I'm scared; this mindfulness thing . . . that you can get is for a few minutes, it's just a few minutes release and peace from that and it's the first time where I stop moving.*" Fostering the ability to be grounded in a decentered awareness of the breath and body makes it possible to be open to unpleasant experience without becoming lost in reaction.

For people with psychosis, moments of decentered awareness often feel calming (Abba et al., 2008): "*[You are] aware of your breathing and that in turn makes you aware of your body and it relaxes*" (Martin). In these moments a person is still aware of the feeling tone of sensations, which can be associated with some stress and tension in the body. It is important to confirm that this does not mean there is anything wrong with the person's mindfulness practice, and to highlight that some sensations, such as images associated with trauma memories, are intrinsically unpleasant. Crucially, in moments of decentered awareness, the person is aware of the unpleasant sensation without avoidance, judgment, or struggle.

Turning toward the Difficult

In mindfulness practice a person chooses to allow psychosis sensations to come fully into awareness. This *turning toward the difficult* (Kabat-Zinn, 2013) is a significant shift for people with psychosis. Ordinarily and understandably many people exhaust themselves in a desperate effort to keep voices, images, thoughts, feelings, and other sensations out of awareness. By grounding themselves in an awareness of the breath and body, they are able, for a few moments and often for the first time, to open awareness and observe psychosis sensations that arise.

Turning toward does not imply looking for or searching out—*we do not encourage people to seek out psychosis experience.* Nor do we ask people to *welcome* unpleasant psychosis sensations, or *invite them in* as is done in some other mindfulness therapies. For most of the people we have worked with, unpleasant psychosis sensations are not welcome. As Marik said, "*I didn't invite them into my head, and I don't want them in there,*" and Faye: "*I haven't invited it into my consciousness, it's invited itself.*" The encouragement is simply to open awareness to include the unpleasant.

Acceptance

Acceptance in the context of mindfulness for psychosis groups combines the meaning of the term as used in mindfulness traditions and the pioneering work of Carl Rogers (1961). Rather than judging psychosis sensations and themselves, a mindful response involves the person accepting that these sensations are happening now, and accepting oneself as someone who is having these experiences in this moment. Acceptance does not mean endorsing or agreeing with the content of a voice, image, or thought. Nor does it mean resignation and defeat in the face of what can seem to be an all-powerful entity. Acceptance is to relate to these sensations and oneself without judgment and so without avoidance and struggle.

A first attribute of acceptance is for the person to accept that *psychosis is part of my experience at this time.* First-person accounts show that when people accept that they hear voices, rather than continuing to fight or resist them, this can be a pivotal step toward recovery (Romme & Escher, 1989). Being part of a group and discovering that others have similar experiences (*universality*; Yalom, 1995) can be transformative:

> "*Accept it. And with the help of the group, you do end up accepting it. Once you've got over that hurdle, I think then you can go forward. If you won't accept the fact that you do have voices and you just fight with them all the time, that's when you just don't go anywhere, you just go round and round.*"—SANDRA

Acceptance has a second important, related quality: Not only are unpleasant voices, images, thoughts, and other sensations a part of my life, *I cannot control them.* This acceptance paves the way for engagement with mindfulness:

> *"The instinct is to push them away, send them away. The problem is it never works. Acceptance is essential—you have to accept that you can't do what you instinctively want to do. It's having faith that they will go even if you don't push them away."*—KAITLIN

The more moments people have of decentered awareness of psychosis experience, the more possible it becomes to accept these sensations as a part of their lives. In moments of decentered awareness, voices and other psychosis experiences are "*deflated*" (Steve) and lose much of their assumed power. When unpleasant sensations are stripped of habitual distressing reactions, acceptance becomes possible, and with acceptance, psychosis loses the power to dominate people's lives.

Acceptance is not a task that can be completed but is an ongoing process. When facilitating mindfulness groups, we keep in mind that everyone will have moments when acceptance of their psychosis and of themselves is not within reach. As Laura put it: "*When I find it hard to accept [these voices] is when I wake in the morning and they are there, straightaway. A person has a right to some peace, some quiet in this world.*" To accept voices first thing in the morning is, for Laura, a challenging daily practice.

Letting Go

When running mindfulness for psychosis groups, it is essential that we understand what it is we are asking people to let go of. All sensations are fleeting, transient experiences: a voice, image, thought, or other sensation arises and then inevitably passes or fades. It is not possible to prolong the sensation itself. Mindfulness is not about letting go of unpleasant experiences, it is about *letting go of habitual reactions* to these psychosis (and other) sensations—the avoiding, judging, worrying, ruminating, and confronting that maintain and escalate distress and disability long after the sensation has passed.

Jane described this as "*Um it's a way of trying to, not get the thoughts to go away, but to stop worrying about them and the anxiety about them,*" and Martin as "*letting go of voices and the meaning of what they're saying, not worrying about what they're saying.*" Richard described this as "*You get a thought coming in and it's a case of down tools,*" and Alison as "*It's like you have to unlearn your responses to these thoughts and feelings. It's like a release for these thoughts and feelings . . . not being tied to fighting with them and struggling with them."* Peter described this simply as "*I remember to try and stay calm when I get a bit of turmoil in my mind.*"

Sometimes a person will notice a specific voice or image as it comes into awareness, and will not react, but this is rare, at least in the first weeks of practicing mindfulness. It is far more usual for letting go to occur when a person catches themselves lost in reacting—that is, people first learn to decenter from reacting and then gently bring their awareness back to the sensations of breathing. As Neil described: "*I'm aware when I lock on to one of these thoughts or ideas or images or whatever has come into my head, when I lock on one of them, and I start following it, I realize I'm doing it and then, whoa, back, refocus.*"

Just as a distressing reaction to psychosis sensations (the left side of the two-circles model) is not a neat sequential process, mindful responding (on the right side) does not describe a predictable series of responses. Mindful responding is not a progression from turning toward the difficult, to accepting, and finally letting go. Rather, these are aspects of an integrated pattern of responding. Like the facets of a glass crystal, each aspect enables and reflects the others.

Fear of Change and Unhelpful Metacognitive Beliefs

While the two-circles model is intended to be a clear and simple description of reacting and responding to unpleasant psychosis sensations, the act of letting go of habitual distressing reactions can feel extremely frightening, and we must not lose sight of this. Kaitlin and Sandra attended one of our first mindfulness groups. Kaitlin saw what she described as bizarre and upsetting images, and heard a malevolent, omnipotent voice. Sandra heard several critical, omnipotent voices that repeatedly threatened her and her family. The following dialogue describes how they felt when they first began to practice mindfulness:

FACILITATOR: I wonder how it felt to begin, for example, to let go of trying to push the voices away, trying to push the images away. How did that feel at first?

KAITLIN: Terrifying—to give up my only way of coping with them, and trust that I'd be OK, that's terrifying. I just felt very vulnerable. It was hard not to just get up and run out of the room.

FACILITATOR: So, terrified, vulnerable, when you began to let go of pushing them away. What did you think might happen if you stopped fighting them?

SANDRA: They'd come back in a different way, even worse. So, in a way if had a choice I'd rather live with the voices like I know them, than have them coming back in a different way, and sort of pushing me sideways. I wouldn't know how to cope.

FACILITATOR: Right, so your fear was that even though it was already really hard, it would get worse—is that right?

SANDRA: Yes, they'd come back even stronger, even more painful.

FACILITATOR: So, it's understandable that even though fighting them wasn't working, you kept doing it, because you were both afraid that if you stopped, it would get even worse.

KAITLIN: Yes, and if they got worse, I'd lose all contact with reality, and that would completely cut me off from my family.

FACILITATOR: Right, so these ways of coping felt like the only way of keeping in contact with reality and staying close to your family.

KAITLIN: It's like I'm far out at sea and I can't swim and you're asking me to let go of my life belt.

Metacognition describes generalized beliefs about our own thinking and mental processes. This incorporates all processes involved in sensory and perceptual experiences, including hearing voices, seeing images, thinking, feeling, bodily sensations, and our overarching sense of self. Kaitlin and Sandra show us how the prospect of change can be terrifying in part because of unhelpful *metacognitive beliefs* regarding the benefits of habitual reactions and feared consequences of responding differently. Sandra describes a version of what is perhaps the single most common unhelpful metacognitive belief regarding voices—that is, "*It is only my struggle and resistance that prevent me from being totally overwhelmed and destroyed.*" These metacognitive beliefs are usually implicit, and need to be drawn out and stated clearly, as illustrated in the dialogue above. Paul spent many hours each day thinking, thinking, thinking about his persecution. One of the factors maintaining this was his metacognitive belief that "*I have to work out what is going on, solve it, it's my best chance of ever being safe and free.*"

Metacognitive Insights

How is it that mindfulness practice can produce lasting, beneficial change? How is it that moments of decentered awareness of transient sensations can change how people experience psychosis, themselves, and their lives? Lasting change occurs when a person gains a new and helpful metacognitive understanding or *metacognitive insight* about their internal experience (Segal, Williams, et al., 2002; Teasdale, 1993). In mindfulness for psychosis groups, the key metacognitive insights relate to new ways of understanding psychosis, distress, well-being, and the self (see Figure 2.2). Metacognitive insights comprise a *generalized* understanding of one's own internal world that emerges *experientially through moments of decentered awareness* of psychosis sensations, and facilitates mindful responding.

If a person says of a single voice, image, or thought, "*That didn't last long,*" this is simply a description of one specific event, whereas if over time they notice that "*Voices and images come into my head and then go, they don't last long,*" this describes a generalized understanding about the nature of sensations and articulates a metacognitive insight that facilitates a shift to mindful responding (the right side of the two-circles model). It is this generalized quality that we seek to draw out in group discussions, to prompt people to broaden learning from specific to wider contexts to promote mindful responding.

Metacognitive insights relate to *one's own internal world.* Consider the belief held by many people with paranoia that "*the world is a dangerous*

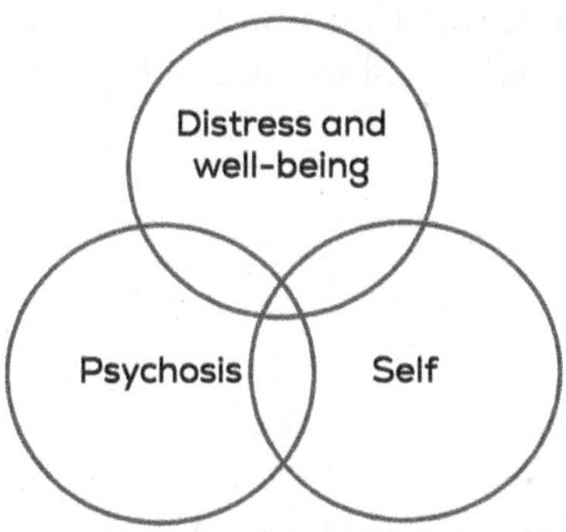

FIGURE 2.2. Focus of metacognitive insights.

place with people who cannot be trusted and want to harm me." While this type of persecutory thinking certainly influences emotion and behavior, it describes the outer world and other people and is therefore not a metacognitive insight. However, if a person with paranoia starts to recognize that "*My beliefs about the world make me scared whenever I meet new people*," they are developing a broad understanding of the nature of their own internal processes that is likely to facilitate mindful responding—a metacognitive insight. In the guided mindfulness practices and the discussions that follow (inquiry), we encourage people to observe and articulate reactions and responses to psychosis sensations, to facilitate metacognitive insights about their internal world.

In mindfulness for psychosis groups, metacognitive insights typically emerge experientially through moments of decentered awareness during guided practices and are then put into words during the subsequent discussion. This contrasts with knowledge or ideas learned from a book or offered by a therapist. While such knowledge or ideas can influence emotion and behavior, it is only when we have closely observed our own mental processes that the *felt sense* of a metacognitive insight emerges.

Through facilitating generalized understanding and experience of individuals' own internal world, we can support people to gain a decentered awareness of their psychosis experiences, and so begin to change their relationship with psychosis and themselves. Table 2.1 describes common unhelpful metacognitive beliefs and helpful metacognitive insights that we listen for and attend to in the groups.[1]

To summarize, in mindfulness for psychosis groups we aim to facilitate moments of decentered awareness, and draw out metacognitive insights about psychosis, suffering, and the self, and in this way support people to change their relationship with both psychosis and themselves.

---

[1]These are examples. Different people will frame these slightly differently and we do not need to get to the wording that fits best for us as facilitators. As in other therapies, these therapeutic insights have more impact if people come to them (with guidance) themselves, and are captured in their own words.

TABLE 2.1. Common Metacognitive Beliefs That Maintain Distressing Reactions, and Metacognitive Insights That Support Mindful Responding

Unhelpful metacognitive beliefs	Helpful metacognitive insights
Distressing reaction	Mindful responding
It is only my struggle and resistance that stop me from being totally overwhelmed and destroyed. I must control my mind.	We can get locked into our minds. All sensations are transient. Reacting is distressing and exhausting. Not reacting is possible and can feel calming, peaceful.
Avoiding	Turning toward the difficult
If I let them in, I'll be overwhelmed and lose control. I can't bear this.	I can step back and observe voices, images, thoughts, and feelings. When I'm grounded in my breath, I can bear psychosis.
Struggling—ruminating, worry, confronting	Letting go
I have to keep struggling, keep fighting, or I'll be overwhelmed. Until I can work this out, solve it, I'll never be free.	I have some choice. When I let go of the struggle, I feel calmer, stronger, more in control.
Judging	Accepting
It's wrong to think, hear, or see these things. Our thoughts and voices reveal who we really are. Bad people have bad thoughts. I am fundamentally different and set apart from other people.	We all have unpleasant thoughts, feelings, and sensations. I cannot control the psychosis and it does not have to control me. Judging creates distress, tension, exhaustion, mental turmoil. When I accept my psychosis and myself, I feel more human. I am fundamentally the same as other people. I am more than the psychosis.

Note. These are illustrative examples; people use different forms of words to convey these beliefs and insights.

3

Mindfulness for Psychosis

A HUMANIZING THERAPEUTIC PROCESS

In the previous chapter, we presented the two-circles model—a conceptual framework contrasting habitual distressing reactions and mindful responding to unpleasant psychosis sensations. In this chapter, we describe the second theory underpinning mindfulness for psychosis: the psychological *process of change* that describes how people move from habitual reacting to mindful responding. This core process of change explains how people with current distressing psychosis learn to relate differently to their psychosis and themselves through mindfulness practice.

We are not suggesting that mindfulness is a cure for psychosis. From a mindfulness perspective, we do not assume there is an illness to cure, rather there is the presence in awareness of typically unpleasant experiences (voices, images, thoughts, confusion, and other sensations) that trigger a set of reactions that create a self-perpetuating, distressed state of mind. With an emphasis on turning toward the difficult, acceptance, and letting go of struggle, mindfulness for psychosis is better understood as enabling people to live well with psychosis, and thereby supporting personal recovery.

Learning to Relate Differently to Psychosis

When we began facilitating mindfulness for psychosis groups, we were genuinely uncertain about how things would unfold. It was one thing to understand conceptually how mindfulness might be helpful, and quite another for people severely disturbed by voices, images, paranoia, and other forms of psychosis, to learn to decenter and respond mindfully, and to do this in a group setting. We were transparent about this with the people who joined the initial groups and evaluated these closely (Abba et al., 2008; Chadwick et al., 2005; Newman-Taylor et al., 2009). Once we began, we were surprised by how willing people were to participate and how open they were to trying the adapted mindfulness. The core mindfulness practice developed specifically for people with psychosis was working well (see Chapter 4), and we were not seeing adverse events, even when people were using this approach over periods of several months.

What also became apparent was how the brief mindfulness practices and linked discussions (inquiry) were enabling people to change how they related to their psychosis experience. Mindfulness for psychosis was possible! Time and again people highlighted the therapeutic value of learning to step back from psychosis experience, let go of reactivity, and relate mindfully to voices, images, thoughts, and other sensations:

> *"If you've got something you can focus on, like your breathing, then it does help, it stops your mind wandering so much."*—RICHARD

> *"Once you're concentrating on your breathing, um well, the idea is that you will be concentrating so much on your breathing it will bring you straight back to the here and now, the chair you're sitting on and the room you're sitting in, at the time of day you're sitting in it. It will bring you all back to that instead of the negative thoughts that come in your head about the past, the present, the future."*—STEVE

> *"Um, it's a way of trying to not get the thoughts to go away but to stop worrying about them and the anxiety about them."*—JANE

Interestingly, this change was not limited to psychosis experience. We observed people applying this process well beyond distressing psychosis. People described how learning to relate mindfully to psychosis was enabling them to discover, or rediscover, a sense of connection with others, moments of joy, and a common humanity; in short, a process of change that was essentially humanizing.

The Core Process of Change

The first 16 people to attend our mindfulness for psychosis groups took part in a qualitative research study to explore their experiences of this therapy (Abba et al., 2008). Verbatim transcripts of in-depth semi-structured interviews were analyzed using *grounded theory* methodology to construct a psychological theory that is rooted in people's own descriptions and interpretations of their direct experiences (Glaser & Strauss, 1967).

People described how at the time of joining a group, they were tyrannized by their psychosis. They felt powerless and frightened, with little personal agency or sense of control. They explained how the psychosis defined them as set apart, abnormal, bad, and worthless. Freeing themselves from this tyranny required them to fundamentally change their relationship with the frequent psychosis experiences that had dominated their life. The three-stage grounded theory (see Figure 3.1) describes how people are able to change their relationship with psychosis—this sits at the heart of the mindfulness for psychosis program.

Stage 1: Stepping Back

A new relationship with psychosis required people to *step back* and observe psychosis experiences, fostering a *decentered awareness*. A first step in this process was for people to gather and anchor their attention by gently observing their breath or body. Focusing gently on breathing and bodily sensations rooted people in the present and established a base from which they might allow unpleasant voices, images, thoughts, and feelings to come fully into awareness. Developing and then practicing this ability to focus gently on the breath and body enabled people to feel safe enough to try opening awareness to include psychosis experience. In this way, each time a person got lost in reacting to their psychosis, they could gently return to this practice of following the flow of the breath or bodily sensations, limiting how far they could be carried away by psychosis.

The first stage of the grounded theory is therefore learning to observe psychosis experience with decentered awareness. People then

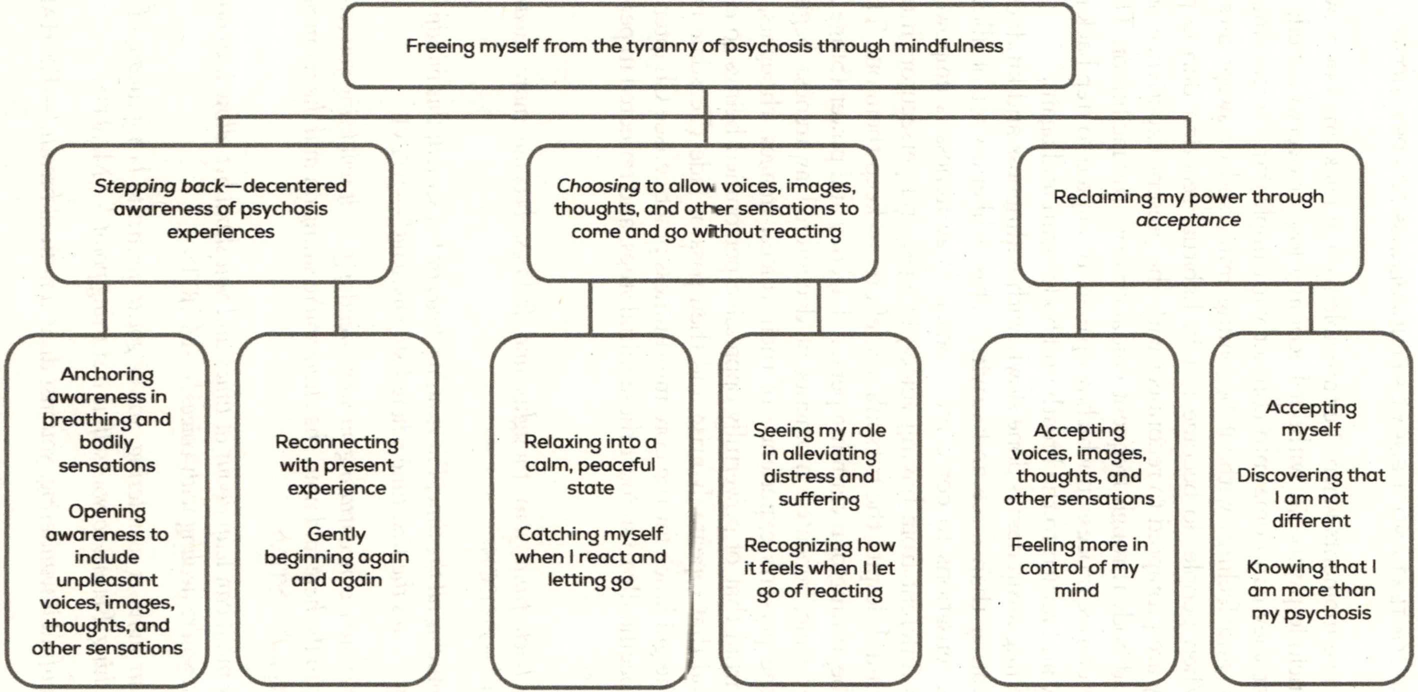

FIGURE 3.1. Grounded theory of learning to respond mindfully to the tyranny of distressing psychosis.

start to have moments when they are able to step back and open awareness to include psychosis, without becoming lost or overwhelmed; they learn that they can come into contact with unpleasant voices, images, thoughts, and feelings without becoming immersed or swept away by them. When people do become lost in habitual reaction during practice, they are prompted to reconnect with the present experience of the breath and body through frequent guidance from the facilitator. This is a gently iterative process in which people are prompted to step back from reactivity and return to the breath and body again and again.

Opening awareness is done slowly with willingness and kindness to oneself, rather than force and striving. This deliberate act of allowing psychosis sensations to come into conscious awareness is empowering and feels different from having voices, images, and persecutors intrude into the mind despite the person's best efforts to keep them out. This is also the beginning of reclaiming personal agency and power (Stage 3).

Over time, repeated moments of decentered awareness begin to change the person's experience of their voices, images, thoughts, and feelings: from that of powerfully oppressive personified beings to *events of the mind* that repeatedly arise and then pass or fade (Teasdale et al., 2002). The guidance for the core mindfulness practice (see Chapter 4) is worded specifically to support these initial steps, and reflected in people's comments:

> *"Step back from your thoughts and feelings, become more aware of them."*—ALISON

> *"I'm moving all the time, I'm running away or I'm scared; this mindfulness thing . . . it's the first time where I stop moving."*—STEVE

> *"Once you're concentrating on your breathing . . . it will bring you straight back to the here and now, the chair you're sitting on and the room you're sitting in."*—STEVE

> *"Your mind can leap about at times and you shouldn't allow it to do that when you're dealing with voices."*—MARTIN

> *"If your mind is wandering, you've got to return to being aware of your breathing. Return to yourself as a starting point."*—MARTIN

> *"If you find it wandering, you just draw a natural breath."*—RICHARD

"[Mindfulness gives] you a physical well-being. Sometimes when you get a bad thought and it gets really stressful, it can affect all the mechanisms in your body and the mindfulness can neutralize those, which makes you feel physically better."—KATHERINE

"At the end of a thought, I'll go back to the breathing."—HANNAH

Stage 2: Choosing to Allow Psychosis to Come and Go without Reacting

The second stage of the grounded theory describes how people begin to release themselves from habitual patterns of reactivity and struggle (the left side of the two-circles model; Chapter 2, Figure 2.1) because they increasingly recognize the effects of reacting and of responding mindfully. This is when people summon the courage to choose to let go of habitual distressing reactions—the avoidance, judgment, rumination, worry, and confrontation—even if just for a moment. Unpleasant psychosis sensations continue to arise, but the person starts to respond differently. This is the stage where people begin to appreciate that mindfulness could give them a different way of living with psychosis.

When people begin to allow psychosis to come and go, it is rare not to react to these sensations. Usually, people begin to react in habitual ways, then catch themselves in the midst of reacting, and then sometimes choose to step back and momentarily let go of their reactivity. Noticing reactions to psychosis while they are happening, and then letting go, enables people to distinguish the unpleasant sensation from their reaction.

Developing decentered awareness of habitual reactivity yields two metacognitive insights regarding *distressing reaction* and *mindful responding*. The first is that "*Reacting is distressing and exhausting.*" As people begin to build their capacity to step back from reactivity, they also discover that "*Not reacting often feels calming and peaceful,*" as tension and stress ease (though mindfulness is not necessarily relaxing). As we saw in Chapter 2, this is a key metacognitive insight, one that challenges the common fear that "*If I stop reacting, I will be overwhelmed by the voices, images, and persecutors*" (an unhelpful metacognitive belief that locks people into reactivity).

These two metacognitive insights—knowing that reacting brings distress, and that letting go of reactivity eases distress—together hold the key to "*Seeing my role in easing my distress*" (see Figure 3.1). When people reflect on both ways of relating to psychosis, they can reach a tipping point when they become disenchanted with habitual reactions, recognizing that these don't work well and are in fact part of the problem, and crucially, a part of the problem over which they can have some control. People then begin to choose to allow psychosis experience to come more frequently and more fully into awareness (Stage 1) and to pass or fade without reacting (Stage 2). Choice is necessary for people to free themselves from the tyranny of psychosis.

In this stage, people start catching themselves in reactivity and choose to let go more frequently. Again, this is a gently iterative process, supported by the core mindfulness practice guidance (see Chapter 4), and reflected in people's comments:

> "*You can either let them go or after 20 minutes you're going to be screaming, breaking windows, throwing your shoes against the wall, banging your fists against the wall. Which one is preferable?*"—MARTIN

> "*Let things come and go . . . If they come, you just let them go and they're not there and you're not fighting with them and you're not struggling with them.*"—ALISON

> "*It's like you have to unlearn your responses to these thoughts and feelings. It's like a release . . . not being tied to fighting with them and struggling with them.*"—ALISON

> "*You don't lose your mind to them.*"—MARTIN

> "*It's as if you've got an override button.*"—KATHERINE

> "*I'm aware when I lock on to one of these thoughts or ideas or images or whatever has come into my head . . . I start following it. I realize I'm doing it and then, whoa, back, refocus.*"—NEIL

> "*Just sort of get fed up with the same old pattern . . . I've been here before, struggling, trying to work them out, fighting.*"—ALISON

> "*Letting go helps, you avoid getting into some ritual that goes on longer than the actual thought or image itself.*"—MICHAEL

> "*There's less fear to it, much less fear . . . [letting go] felt really much safer to do that than to go into it and to run with it.*"—STEVE

Stage 3: Acceptance and Reclaiming Power

The tyranny of psychosis comes in large part from the way voices and perceived persecutors are seemingly omniscient (all seeing) and omnipotent (all powerful), exerting power and control over the person. In the final stage of the grounded theory, people reclaim their power through acceptance of psychosis and themselves.

As people become more able to *step back and observe* unpleasant sensations with decentered awareness (Stage 1), and to *choose how to respond* (Stage 2), people describe an emerging sense of being more in control of their mind and their life. People come to recognize the twin metacognitive insights that "*I cannot control the psychosis*" and that "*Psychosis does not have to control me.*" Gradually, people start to realize that by stepping back and not reacting, the psychosis has less power and control than they had believed.

Perceiving psychosis experiences with decentered awareness, without the frenetic striving and stress of the person's own reactivity, has the effect of *deflating* voices, images, thoughts, and other sensations that can now be experienced more simply as they are: as unpleasant, intrusive experiences that come into awareness and then pass or fade. This makes accepting psychosis a possibility. At the outset of the process, the idea of accepting psychosis is inconceivable, whereas having experienced moments of decentered awareness, accepting psychosis sensations stripped of the person's reaction now becomes a possibility. As psychosis experience deflates, and as people no longer focus all their attention and energy on reacting, they begin to feel more in control of their own mind, can connect with valued aspects of themselves, and are able to engage more fully in their lives. Psychosis no longer defines them, and they know from direct experience, "*I am more than my psychosis.*"

This final step in the process is rooted in a deep and grounded self-acceptance. As with all parts of the theory, the process is supported not only through mindfulness practice and linked discussion but through being part of a group. Self-acceptance is supported when people recognize that others have similar experiences (universality) and are accepted by the others in the group (cohesion and belonging). Self-acceptance is supported by people noticing their common humanity with others, including the group facilitators, and no longer feeling set apart, different, and alien, as a growing sense of humanization unfolds:

"I can accept the thoughts that come into my head as opposed to struggle with them."—HANNAH

"Let the voices happen and you'll find out they meant nothing anyway . . . If you've got voices controlling you, try and just let it and then you'll find out that it didn't control you after all. It's just a voice."—GARETH

"It's that not judging what's going through your head, it's just accepting it as what it is, not worried about vindictive voices, or whatever, it's just accepting it, that's the way it is. No right, no wrong."—NEIL

"If I'm judging the thoughts I have, I can judge myself as good or bad. If I'm not judging, it makes me feel better about myself."—SALLY

"It's like today's session, I said my head was like a newsreel and that was OK, and there's a load of different images, voices, and things in my head and that was OK, whereas before this kind of stuff was happening I was fighting against it, thinking, 'No, this is wrong, this is wrong,' . . . It's a completely new way of looking at it, you know, of accepting it instead of fighting against it nonstop, worrying about it, thinking, 'Oh my God, another relapse.' Just accept it . . . When I'm accepting everything the way it's meant to be at that particular moment in time, then things are OK, and I feel OK."—NEIL

". . . makes you feel whole. You grow stronger with it."—ALISON

"It's improved me as a person."—KATHERINE

"Acceptance that perhaps I'm no different . . . listening to someone else's experience, who I regard as so-called normal, or whatever, and that their experience was the same, that helped me accept a big chunk about myself. I've thought that basically I'm not wrong, that I'm quite acceptable."—NEIL

How Do Individuals Embody the Theory?

The core process of change in mindfulness for psychosis, described by the grounded theory (Abba et al., 2008), is an iterative, nonlinear developmental process. People move back and forth between stages, and in and out of connecting with this process. Everyone attending the groups continues to have moments of reactivity, lost in struggle with familiar, habitual patterns, and self-dehumanization (the left side of the two-circles model). Moreover, the entire process does not have a set end point. Accepting psychosis and the self can deepen over time, but ebbs and flows for everyone. Furthermore, the theory describes a humanizing therapeutic process that occurs within an ever-changing set of life circumstances and conditions. What is required to embody the principles underlying the process of becoming mindful of psychosis therefore also shifts from one week to the next. As facilitators, our role is to create the conditions for mindful responding as best we can.

We are also not suggesting that all individuals engage with and embody the three stages equally. As with all mindfulness-based interventions, indeed, as with all therapeutic work, people vary in how much they change. What deepens a person's engagement in each stage in the theory is not only the quality and quantity of moments of decentered awareness but the extent to which these moments lead to helpful metacognitive insights. It is our experience that most people attending the groups experience all three stages to some degree. Indeed, it could be argued that in any moment of responding mindfully, all three stages are present, even if largely implicit.

Coda to Part I

As you reach the end of Part 1 of this book, we take a moment to reflect on what we have introduced so far. Our intention has been to convey a sense of excitement and possibility about the potential that mindfulness for psychosis presents.

Chapter 1 set out the challenge and urgency that led us to develop mindfulness for psychosis. In Chapter 2 we described a framework for understanding distressing reactivity and mindful responding. This forms the basis for understanding how mindfulness can be applied in any given moment to unpleasant psychosis sensations, introducing the concepts of decentered awareness (stepping back from internal experience), acceptance in this context, and metacognitive beliefs and insights (that lock people into distressing reaction or enable mindful responding). Here in Chapter 3, we have argued that the benefits of mindfulness for psychosis can go beyond how people relate to psychosis experience, framing this as a humanizing therapeutic process that supports people to become themselves and lead their lives more fully.

Our focus throughout this book is to describe a theory and therapy that can be used by clinicians and facilitators thinking of running mindfulness groups for people with psychosis. We hope Part 1 provides the conceptual clarity needed to empower you to bring a sure-footedness and gently confident approach into the therapy room.

We developed the conceptual framework, combining the two-circles model and core process of change (based on the grounded theory), over time as we led the early groups, evaluated these, and talked with many people with psychosis about this approach and their personal recovery. If there is a danger in our presenting all this at the outset, it is that this might create expectations of what *should* be happening in mindfulness groups, and might lead you to *strive to make this happen.* It is important that we ourselves are as mindful as we can be when we lead these groups, and as best we can, let go of the striving that risks pushing people along an expected path or process to a particular end point. The essence of mindfulness for psychosis can be lost, and the approach denatured, if we become lost in striving and trying to move or push people toward a predetermined goal that we have in mind.

We say more on this in later chapters; for now, suffice to say it is also important for our own well-being that we do our best to be mindful ourselves and allow things to unfold as they will. Our task is to create the conditions that support people to develop a mindful relationship with psychosis experiences, greater self-acceptance, and self-humanization, as best we can. We encourage you to follow the detailed guidance here, trust the therapeutic process, and trust the people in the group as they recover from the tyranny of psychosis, as best they can.

II

Mindfulness in Practice

4

The Core Mindfulness Practice and Moments of Mindfulness in Daily Life

Many people with psychosis begin the program fearing they will not be able to *do mindfulness*. Certainly, they face significant challenges. Mindfulness practices and group discussions are punctuated by frequent omnipotent, malevolent voices and images, fears about perceived persecutors, confusion, self-doubt and despair, and other unpleasant feelings, urges, memories, and sensations. Tiredness is common, as is anxiety about traveling and meeting new people. Psychiatric medications have side effects that can make practice challenging. Against this backdrop, it is essential that mindfulness does not become one more thing that people come to believe they are getting wrong, cannot do, or are failing.

These challenges and risks of anticipated failure led us to aspire to introduce mindfulness in a way that was true to the core elements of the practice, while giving people every possibility of being able to connect with, learn, and benefit from this approach. This led us to develop the *10-minute core mindfulness practice* for people with psychosis, which is used twice every session and lays the foundation for people to learn to relate mindfully to psychosis in the groups and in daily life.

In our program there is no requirement for home practice, though this is encouraged and supported with audio recordings (see Chapter 8 for more detail). We accept and appreciate whatever home practice is possible. This pragmatic position embodies acceptance of the challenges of living with psychosis and minimizes the risk of people thinking that they are failing or letting others down. To help embed mindfulness in daily life, we also introduce three prompts to support people to practice relating mindfully to pleasant, unpleasant, and neutral sensations day-to-day and moment-to-moment.

The Core Mindfulness Practice

The core mindfulness practice for people with psychosis lasts approximately 10 minutes. This is in contrast to sometimes lengthy traditional practices, and other secular applications of up to 20 or 45 minutes. For most people, voices, images, thoughts, and other unpleasant psychosis sensations are so frequent that 10 minutes is ample time to learn to observe and recognize habitual reactions, and to explore stepping back and relating mindfully to psychosis—that is, to become experientially familiar with both sides of the two-circles model (see Chapter 2, Figure 2.1). A relatively brief core mindfulness practice also minimizes the risk of people either struggling to stay with the guidance until the end, or finding this draining and aversive, which in turn risks perceived failure.

Having two practices each session means that when people find the first "*didn't work*," or they "*couldn't do it*," there is an opportunity to discuss this during the inquiry and have a different experience in the second practice. Having two practices also helps facilitators; if some elements of the guidance are missed in the first, these can be included in the second, as well as weaving in one or two important points that have emerged during the session to that point.

When guiding a core mindfulness practice, we refer explicitly to voices, images, paranoia, and other forms of psychosis experienced by individuals in the group, using the same gentle tone as when referring to other sensations. This implicitly normalizes psychosis experiences and begins subtly to question the omnipotence attributed to voices and perceived persecutors.

We avoid silences of longer than 20–30 seconds. Hearing facilitators' voices anchors people during practice and reduces the likelihood of them becoming lost in psychosis and reactivity. However, constant guidance is also avoided because this can create sensory overload for people with frequent intrusive voices, images, and thoughts, which often continue throughout mindfulness practices. The core mindfulness practice for people with psychosis therefore seeks to balance frequent guidance and short silences.

The Core Practice: Structure and Focus of Decentered Awareness

The core mindfulness practice combines *focused* and *open* (*choiceless*) awareness—two aspects of traditional mindfulness practices (Chadwick, 2006). Both are forms of *decentered awareness*, and differ in what is being observed, though not in the quality of awareness. Focused awareness rests attention on a particular place (e.g., on the breath), whereas open awareness involves observing whatever is in the foreground of the attentional field. It is helpful to think of the core mindfulness practice in terms of an opening, middle, and closing phase (see Figure 4.1).

The opening phase begins with establishing *focused decentered awareness*. The guidance gently encourages people to focus their attention on areas of the body, and then narrows in on sensations of breathing. In the middle phase, the guidance prompts people to *open their attention* to all sensations that come into awareness, including voices, images, thoughts, feelings, memories, sounds, and bodily sensations. Awareness

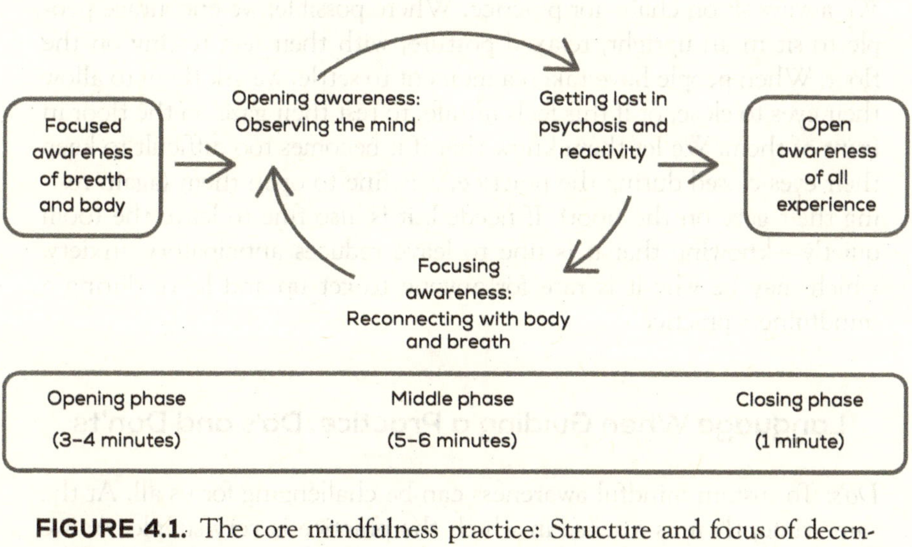

FIGURE 4.1. The core mindfulness practice: Structure and focus of decentered awareness.

stays with whatever is in the foreground without trying to *pull* attention back to the breathing.

During the middle phase people repeatedly lose decentered awareness and become lost in psychosis and distressing reaction. The guidance prompts people to notice and let go of moments of avoidance, struggle, and judgment, reestablish awareness of the sensations of breathing for a few moments, and then once more to open their attention to all experiences that arise. With practice, people may start to catch themselves in reactivity unprompted, let go, and bring themselves back to the sensations of the breath and wider awareness, reestablishing decentered awareness independently. This *beginning again and again* to reconnect with the breath and sensations as they arise, with a gentle and kind attitude, is an important part of changing the relationship with psychosis and the self.

As we enter the closing phase, the guidance lets people know there is 1 minute left, and encourages open awareness of all experiences, whether pleasant, unpleasant, or neutral. The practice then ends by prompting people to bring their awareness back to the room, and gently open their eyes when ready.

Preparation for Practice

We always sit on chairs for practice. Where possible, we encourage people to sit in an upright, relaxed posture, with their feet resting on the floor. When people have taken a moment to settle, we ask them to allow their eyes to close, or if this feels unsafe, to rest their gaze on the floor in front of them. We let them know that if it becomes too difficult to keep their eyes closed during the practice, it is fine to open them (again resting their gaze on the floor). If needed, it is also fine to leave the room quietly—knowing that it is fine to leave reduces anticipatory anxiety, which may be why it is rare for anyone to get up and leave during a mindfulness practice.

Language When Guiding a Practice: Do's and Don'ts

Do's: To sustain mindful awareness can be challenging for us all. At the same time, there is a sense in which the practice is very simple. As we often say, "*All we are doing here is sitting down, closing our eyes, and as best we can, noticing what we experience and how we react.*" We also use simile, though sparingly; it can be useful when guiding people to allow voices, images, thoughts, and other sensations to come into awareness and pass or fade, "*like clouds in the sky,*" "*like images on a screen,*" or "*like leaves on a stream.*" When guiding a practice, we recommend using language that is:

- Simple and down-to-earth
- Gentle and kind (e.g., "*gently bringing your awareness back*")
- Balanced and steady in tone and warmth
- Accepting (e.g., frequent use of "*as best we can*")
- Normalizing of difficulty and facilitative of universality (e.g., "*we all get lost in this way*")

Don'ts: We do not encourage people to visualize *placing* unpleasant sensations on a river or equivalent. This does not work well with voices and images, can reinforce the misconception that the aim is to get rid of these experiences or empty the mind, and might give the impression that the sensation would not have passed of its own accord (which all sensations do). Guidance neither needs nor benefits from language that is complex, clever, or spiritual. We recommend avoiding:

- The term *body scan*, which can arouse fear and paranoia in people with psychosis
- Metaphor that might sound concerning or bizarre—for example, talk of moving the mind, parts of the body dissolving, or breathing in and out from different places in the body such as the head and toes
- Referring to voices, images, thoughts, or feelings as *guests* or *visitors*
- Talk of *welcoming* unpleasant experiences, which can be immediately invalidating
- Spiritual language and phrases
- Any suggestion that practice will or should lead to relaxation, which risks people thinking they have failed or got it wrong if they don't feel relaxed
- Talk of creating a *safe space* or a time that is set aside just for them—again, this risks a sense of failure for people who experience voices, paranoia, and other psychosis sensations much of the day every day.

People with psychosis are individuals and these cautions will not apply to all but in a group setting it is better to err on the side of caution.

The Core Mindfulness Practice: An Overview

The first practice in each session follows a standard text or script. Before you lead others in this core practice, it's worth taking time to consider the specific components of the script. In what follows here we look closely at those components and offer explanatory comments. (For your convenience, Appendix 9.1 has the script for this practice, without the commentary.) While the second practice also closely follows the flow and sequence of the script, facilitators may weave in one or two points to emphasize the focus for the session or pick up on relevant points discussed during inquiry after the first practice (the opening phase can be shortened slightly if necessary to create time for this).

Script for the Core Mindfulness Practice

Opening Phase

Core mindfulness script	Commentary
1. Let's start by taking a moment to sit comfortably in the chair, sitting in an upright, relaxed position with your feet resting on the floor. If it feels comfortable, allow your eyes to close, or if you prefer, rest your gaze on the floor in front of you. It is easy to get locked in our minds, lost in thinking, so we begin mindfulness by bringing our awareness to our bodies. It can help to bring our awareness to a point of contact, so if you can, gently bring your awareness to the soles of your feet on the floor. Really connect with the sensations in this place in your body—maybe notice feelings of temperature or pressure. Maybe warmth or cold.	"*It is easy to get locked in our minds, lost in thinking, so we begin mindfulness by bringing our awareness to our bodies*"—this opening phrase incorporates an important metacognitive insight ("*we can get locked into our minds*") and rationale for grounding awareness initially in the body and sensations of breathing. ". . . *bring your awareness to the soles of your feet on the floor*"—decentered awareness of the soles of the feet is grounding both literally and figuratively and so is used in each practice.
2. Sometimes, if we really connect with the sensations in the soles of our feet, we can notice tingling sensations that move around and come and go. We can see how nothing stays in awareness for long.	"*We can see how nothing stays in awareness for long*"—decentered awareness of bodily sensations arising and passing supports the metacognitive insight that "*all sensations are transient.*"

3. Now gently bringing your awareness up into your legs. Just noticing whatever sensations are present right now in this part of your body, maybe noticing the pressure of the chair, or the feeling of clothing against your skin. Don't worry if you can't notice any sensations in a part of your body; this is quite normal. Now, moving your awareness to your upper body: your torso, arms, and hands. Just noticing whatever sensations are happening right now in this moment. And across your shoulders. We often carry a lot of tension in our shoulders; if you become aware that your shoulders are tense, seeing if it is possible to relax them a little. Bringing your awareness to your face, scalp, and inside your mouth.	For many people, a decentered awareness of present-moment sensations is more accessible when focused on bodily sensations rather than psychosis experiences. The guidance supports decentered awareness of broad areas of the body and not a fine-grained body scan. We omit reference to the pelvic area, which may increase self-consciousness unhelpfully. Prior to mindfulness practice, many people are unaware of how their bodies feel—for example, not realizing how tired or tense they are. Noticing this often generates an enthusiasm for mindfulness. Over the course of the 8 weeks, mindfulness practice begins to establish generalized bodily awareness and to reverse any dissociation from bodily experience—for example, following neglect or trauma.
4. Now bring your awareness gently to the sensations in your body as you breathe in and as you breathe out. Find that place in your body where you can really notice the sensations as you breathe in and breathe out, where it's comfortable for you to rest your awareness. This might be noticing the rise and fall of your tummy or chest as you breathe in and out, or you	Awareness of the sensations of breathing is also awareness of the body. Sometimes minor variation in the guidance can reflect this—for example: "*Continuing to focus on our bodies, let's now bring our attention to the sensations of breathing.*"

may prefer to focus on the tips of your nostrils, noticing the sensations as the cooler air comes in and the slightly warmer air comes out.	
5. We are not trying to change or control our breathing in any way. Mindfulness is about experiencing things just as they are. So, as best we can, experiencing one in-breath from its beginning to end just as it is, one out-breath from its beginning to end just as it is.	
Middle Phase	
Note. The middle phase typically has slightly longer gaps between points in the guidance, lengthening this phase of the practice.	
6. We are not trying to force our attention to stay on the breathing. What we all find is that our awareness moves naturally to other things: sounds, thoughts, voices, images, memories, worries, judgments, feelings. For these few minutes, if we can, we allow each of these sensations to come fully into awareness, and then allow them to pass or fade into the background, without reacting to them. Then each time we allow our awareness gently to return and rest again in the sensations of breathing.	This guidance rejects the idea that participants should try to hold their attention on their breathing. Psychosis experiences are named in a simple, neutral tone that ascribes them no more importance than other thoughts, feelings, and sensations. This helps normalize voices, images, and perceived persecutors, and implicitly questions their omnipotence and special status. *"For these few minutes if we can we allow . . ."* encourages opening of awareness while recognizing how difficult and frightening it can be to let go of habitual reactions to psychosis experience.

7. You may find that difficult voices, images, thoughts, feelings, and other sensations come back again a few moments later. This is what happens. As best we can, each time we patiently allow difficult voices, images, thoughts, and feelings to come fully into awareness and then to pass or fade, without getting lost or caught up in them, without thinking about them or trying to work them out. In the spaces between the voices, images, thoughts, and other sensations, allowing our awareness to gently return to rest in the sensations of breathing.	This (and Point 6) conveys the essence of open awareness by talking of "*. . . not trying to force our attention to stay on the breathing*" and "*. . . each time we patiently allow difficult voices, images, thoughts, and feelings to come fully into awareness.*" This also guards against the common tendency to try and wrest awareness away from prominent psychosis experience and pull it back to the breath, which creates tension and a sense of failure or defeat. "*In the spaces between the voices, images, thoughts, and other sensations, allowing our awareness gently to return to rest in the sensations of breathing*"—importantly, this reminds us that as voices and other sensations pass or fade into the background, an awareness of the sensations of breathing continues to function as an anchor for our attentional focus, even during open awareness.
8. Often, we find we have been lost, maybe struggling with voices, caught up in rumination or worry. We all get lost like this. There is no need to judge yourself. When this happens, as best we can, we notice how it feels in the body, how it feels emotionally, to let go of this struggle and reconnect with the sensations of breathing. Just resting our awareness in the sensations as we breathe in and as we breathe out.	Here, we are normalizing the experience of getting lost or caught up in reactivity and losing decentered awareness. Group members have told us how valuable it is to hear that facilitators also experience this. The universality of getting lost is offered as a basis for letting go of self-criticism and judgment.

9. Remembering that we are not trying to get rid of voices, images, thoughts, and feelings. We are not trying to create an empty mind. We are practicing being with difficult voices, images, thoughts, and sensations in a different way—allowing them to come fully into awareness and pass or fade without having to react, without having to struggle or fight or analyze.	This addresses the most pervasive misunderstanding about mindfulness: that the goal is to empty the mind, and get rid of difficult voices, images, thoughts, and feelings.
10. If even once you are able to allow a difficult voice, thought, or image to come fully into awareness and pass or fade without reacting, if you can do this even once, notice how that feels in your body, emotionally, in your mind.	Here (and in Point 8), we are directing people's attention to how it feels to let go of reacting, and to allow voices and other psychosis sensations to come and go without reaction. This draws attention to key material for subsequent group discussion (inquiry) about distressing reactivity and mindful responding (the two-circles model).
Closing Phase	
11. For the last minute, as best we can, really being open to whatever sensations arise, whether pleasant or unpleasant or neutral. Allowing all experiences to come fully into awareness and then pass or fade without reacting.	The closing phase encourages open awareness of all experience. Letting people know that there is just 1 minute left increases the likelihood of people finishing the practice with some moments of decentered awareness.
12. When you are ready, gently open your eyes and settle back into the room.	We favor a simple invitation to open the eyes rather than a meditation bell in mindfulness for psychosis groups in secular health care settings.

Applying Mindfulness in Daily Life

We encourage people to use the core mindfulness practice every day. Some people are able to do this, and others do not. Even with little or no home practice, two guided practices each session lays the foundation for relating mindfully to psychosis and bringing mindful awareness into daily life.

To build on this, we introduce three prompts for *mindful moments*—to apply mindfulness in daily life. These are not guided practices and are not time-tabled into the day. The three prompts broadly align with the earlier categorization of the *feeling tone* of sensory experience as pleasant, unpleasant, or neutral (see Chapter 2).

We have suggested when to introduce these prompts in the group manual (see Chapters 8–12). However, often they emerge spontaneously during discussion of mindfulness over the previous week, and we encourage facilitators to be flexible and willing to introduce these when members of a particular group are likely to benefit.

Prompting Moments of Mindfulness: "Checking In with Ourselves"

During discussion and at the initial check-in each session, people often report spontaneous moments of mindfulness during the week. Initially, these typically focus on *neutral sensations* or situations, perhaps making a cup of tea, taking a bus, or waiting in a shopping line. As facilitators, we are interested in these spontaneous moments of mindfulness, and listen for, encourage, and reinforce these.

When the situation is fairly neutral, a simple *checking in with ourselves* can be a helpful prompt to decenter, and can be facilitated simply—for example: "*That's great. These moments of mindfulness in daily life are really important. Just taking a few moments to drop into the body, be aware of our bodies, draw a couple of natural breaths. Whenever we remember, taking just a few moments to check in with ourselves builds a new mindful habit.*"

The key to checking in with ourselves when things are neutral is remembering to choose to be mindful for just a few moments and then tune into the sensations in the body and the flow of sensations as we breathe in and breathe out. A reminder on a phone or a card in a purse or wallet can help.

Prompting Moments of Mindfulness: Opening to Moments of Joy and Connection

Often by Session 2, again during the initial session check-in, someone comments on a mindful moment linked to a *pleasant sensation*. This can result in a deep sense of joy and connection. Faye described one such moment when walking to her second group session. As was often the case, she was lost in her thoughts, feeling distressed by malevolent voices and financial worries. She glanced up at a cherry tree in blossom and immediately turned away and continued walking, head down, again lost in fear and worry. She then remembered the group, stopped, and looked over at the tree. She walked back and sat down under the tree on a carpet of fallen blossoms and grass. For a few minutes Faye simply sat and allowed herself to be aware of the smell, the feel of the ground and sunshine on her skin, the light, the sounds. She told the group it was the happiest she had felt in years.

This is more than simply an experience of pleasure. This is a moment of direct, embodied, and joyful connection with the world around us. Opening to moments of joy and connection shows how mindfulness applies to all experience, not only the unpleasant, and increases motivation to embed mindfulness in daily life. Sharing such moments can be nourishing for everyone present and directly supports all four interrelated group factors that underpin engagement and change in mindfulness for psychosis groups: universality, group cohesion, hope, and being myself more fully (these are discussed in Chapter 6).

If opening to moments of joy and connection has not come up spontaneously, we introduce this prompt in Session 2 during the opening check-in: "*We want to mention today that we can be mindful of all experience, not just the difficult stuff. Has anyone had any moments over the last week when they took a few seconds to really connect with something pleasant or joyful? Maybe with a friend or a pet, listening to music, or being in nature?*"

Inviting reflection on opportunities for joy and connection in everyday life typically prompt some people to recall recent examples and the impact on their mood and well-being, and others to tune into the possibility of such moments. Facilitators might share an example themselves, illustrating how an everyday situation can bring a sense of joy and connection—for example: "*I'd been feeling tired so was thinking about canceling a plan to meet up with friends but didn't want to let them down.*

Later that evening, when we were all laughing together, I noticed a sense of shared joy and connection, and how fulfilling this felt." By describing occasions with others, when absorbed in a valued pursuit, or in nature, we can model noticing mindful moments of connection and joy, emphasizing that it is the quality of direct connection with what is around us that matters.

Reflective discussion in Sessions 2 and 3 highlight how we all miss many potential moments of joy and connection when we are lost in distressing reactions such as avoidance, rumination, and judgment. For some, this adds to the motivation to let go of habitual reactivity. We encourage people to look for such opportunities in daily life and are interested in examples brought in subsequent sessions:

> *"These little moments of joy in life are so important. It's important to see them, and it's important to value them."*—JAY

Prompting Moments of Mindfulness: Aware, Breathe, and Choose (ABC) When Facing Unpleasant Sensations

By Session 3, people are starting to feel able to let go of reactions to difficult internal sensations, and many are already generalizing this to stressful situations in daily life. From Session 3, we prompt people to *step back* and use mindfulness when faced with unpleasant or stressful events day-to-day. Again, a key issue here is to remember to use mindfulness at times of heightened arousal and stress. A simple ABC mnemonic can be helpful here:

- Be *aware*—stop, step back, notice what's happening right now—around us, in the body
- *Breathe*—drop the attention into the body and *draw a natural breath*
- *Choose* how to respond—what will be most useful to me right now?

The sequence shown in Figure 4.2 mirrors the flow of the core mindfulness practice, and maps on to the first two stages of the central process of change (see Chapter 3). This can then become part of the weekly opening check-in from Session 4 onward, and can be immediately impactful. For example:

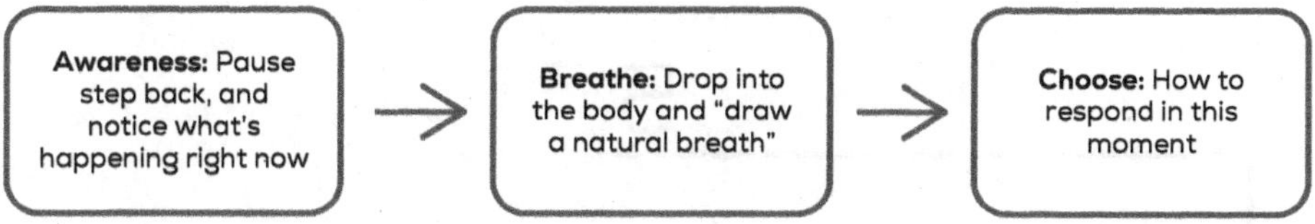

FIGURE 4.2. Prompting mindfulness in daily life: Stepping back from psychosis (aware, breathe, choose [ABC]).

> *"Yes, I've got a choice. When I'm feeling desperate, I can pause, take a breath, come back to myself. I've done it a few times now—just pause and take a deep breath and come back to myself. I need to remember to choose to do it but it's possible!"*—PAUL

5

Inquiry

VALIDATING, BUILDING UNIVERSALITY, AND GUIDING DISCOVERY

In the previous chapters we discussed how mindfulness can enable people to free themselves from the tyranny of psychosis by fostering an alternative relationship with voices, images, thoughts, and other sensations moment-to-moment—learning to let these experiences come and go, cultivating an acceptance of psychosis and themselves. This change in relationship arises from a combination of mindfulness practice and inquiry. Mindfulness practice and inquiry work together and are of equal importance; it is typically during inquiry that learning from experiential practice can be articulated and fully realized.

In mindfulness groups for people with psychosis, inquiry refers to all periods of reflective discussion. This includes the opening conversations when people share mindfulness-related experiences since the previous session, dialogue immediately following guided practices, discussion of psychoeducational material, and drawing together key learning toward the end of each session.

Trusting and Empowering the Group: Allowing Inquiry to Flow

How we facilitate inquiry matters. It has long been recognized that having too little session structure in groups for people with psychosis can be anxiety provoking and untherapeutic (cf. Yalom, 1995). It can also be anxiety provoking and untherapeutic when facilitators impose too much structure and control. For example, a *turn-taking* approach in which facilitators systematically work their way around the room, asking each person in turn broadly the same questions, is unhelpful; anxiety typically mounts for those awaiting their turn, and people's replies tend to conform to previous answers to the same question. Additionally, benefits of *group reflection* are likely to be lost and opportunities for learning greatly reduced. Striking a therapeutic balance of structure and open inquiry depends on our willingness to trust and empower the group. As facilitators, we bring our own concerns and anxieties, which can interfere with this. Chapter 13 offers guidance for facilitators who notice an understandable (but unhelpful) urge to impose a tight structure and control over group sessions to manage their own worries.

In mindfulness for psychosis groups, we seek to facilitate inquiry that flows freely at its own pace and rhythm, using only light-touch guidance to maintain focus. This can be done by asking open questions and offering reflections to the group, then allowing people to choose when to speak—that is, trusting people to join in the conversation when ready. This also means that as facilitators we do not jump in too quickly if no one responds immediately, as this closes down opportunities for participation and learning. Allowing brief silences of up to about 10–15 seconds (which is longer than we may think!) is usually sufficient for people to speak if they wish. Facilitators respond to important points as they arise, with reflections, summaries, and questions to avoid longer silences. This style of facilitation conveys trust in the group and feedback suggests that people find this approach validating and empowering. Occasionally a group may struggle initially to establish discussion among group members. If this happens, it can help to begin one or two periods of inquiry by asking people first to reflect in pairs for a couple of minutes before opening the discussion to the whole group; doing this once or twice has always been sufficient to establish more free-flowing group reflection.

Balancing Inquiry with an Individual and with the Group

When guiding discovery, we can either stay focused on a discussion with one person (*vertical* exploration), or we can widen the discussion to include others in the group (*horizontal* exploration)—both are important. Not staying with an individual long enough risks missed opportunities for learning. Staying too long with one person risks making them feel exposed or put on the spot, and the group disengaging. Opening inquiry to the group brings the benefit of drawing on others' experiences and perspectives, keeps the group engaged, and actively builds universality and group cohesion. Balancing individual and group exploration is a key skill in facilitating inquiry. For example:

- Voices—"*When you stopped fighting and came back to your breathing, the voices faded away* (summary). *That's really interesting. I wonder, what does that tell us about the voices' power over you?*" (vertical exploration)
- Images—"*So, it sounds as if today you were able to step back and let the images come and go, you didn't need to block them out* (summary). *I'm wondering, is there anything you've learned about yourself from this experience?*" (vertical exploration)
- Paranoia/grandiosity—"*So, it started when you heard your neighbor laughing. The laughter lasted just a few seconds, but you spent the whole afternoon worrying that they'd been laughing at you, and the more you worried, the worse you felt—is that right?*" (summary). [To the group:] "*I wonder, what can we learn from this about our understandable reactions to these difficult experiences?*" (horizontal exploration)
- Reacting—"*I think what you're saying is important. For a few moments you were able to let go of reacting. You found that when you stepped back, you felt better. Over the last 2 weeks, others have noticed this, too.*" [To the group:] "*What is the impact of reacting all the time to difficult thoughts, voices, or images?*" or "*What does it tell us about how it feels to step back and let go of reacting?*" (horizontal exploration)

Disclosure

When facilitating enquiry, we communicate the importance of people sharing only as much as feels comfortable, and we say that there is no requirement to share the content of difficult thoughts, voices, and images. We might say, "There is no need to tell us about the detail of the voices and images if this is uncomfortable. What we focus on here is the impact these experiences have on us—how we feel and how we react, and how it feels if we can pause, step back, and allow them to come and go without reacting. Only share as much as you're comfortable sharing." In practice, facilitators need to say this not only at the start of the first enquiry in Session 1, but give one or two reminders over subsequent sessions.

Aims and Methods of Inquiry

Inquiry is more than the act of talking as a group. It is not simply a time for people to describe their experiences following a mindfulness practice. While inquiry typically begins with facilitators guiding participants to describe what they noticed during the practice, it is important not to get stuck here (e.g., repeatedly asking "*And what happened next?*" or "*And what did you notice then?*"). Rather, we seek to move reasonably swiftly from individuals' description of direct experience over the previous few minutes of practice, to reflective group discussion focused on *analyzing*, *synthesizing*, and *learning* from these observations, to support mindful responding—that is, to draw out metacognitive insights that enable people to step back from psychosis experiences, let sensations come and go without reaction, and reclaim a sense of autonomy and control through acceptance (see Chapter 4).

The three main methods used to facilitate inquiry are *validation*, *building universality*, and *guiding discovery*, all of which are based on active listening (Rogers & Farson, 1957). When we engage in active listening, we are focused on understanding the other person's experience, feelings, and perspective, and we use reflections, summaries, and questions that help us do this. To sustain active listening requires that as facilitators we monitor our own feelings and reactions during inquiry and, as best we can, step back from any that might pull us away from focusing on the group members—for example, worries about running the group, rehearsing what comes next, or feeling responsible for people benefiting from the program. We recommend that facilitators take a moment prior to starting a session to commit, as best we can, to being fully present for the group members, and focused on understanding their experiences and perspectives. We often need to reset this intention during the session when we realize we have been lost in our own reactions.

Of these three methods of inquiry, validation usually comes first, then either building universality or guiding discovery of metacognitive insights. For example, if a person describes feeling defeated by powerful, abusive voices during a mindfulness practice, we might first validate their sense of defeat (e.g., "*It sounds like you felt utterly defeated by these voices*"). We might then either open to the wider group to explore if others have had similar experiences and build universality (e.g., "*It can understandably be devastating for many of you to have voices, images, and thoughts intrude into your mind every hour of every day*"), or stay with the person to facilitate metacognitive insight (e.g., "*Were there any moments, however fleeting, when you were able to step back and notice the voices without reacting?*" . . . "*And what did that feel like?*" . . . "*And what do you make of that?*"). The sequence is flexible; active listening allows us to start by validating what is key to the person in that moment, and then draw out common experience, or learning, or both.

Validating Experience

Validation involves recognizing and accepting a person's experience, without judgment or blame. Validation is particularly important for people with psychosis who face high levels of stigma from our wider society, have often lost trust in their own judgment, and fear they no longer make sense to other people (O'Brien-Venus et al., 2024), as described by John (see Chapter 1) who told his best friend about his voices and images: "*She told me that I was mad, that no such things existed, and stopped being my friend. It really broke me.*"

When validating distress, trauma, and struggle, it is important to balance this with connection among group members and hope for recovery. During periods of inquiry, we seek to achieve this balance by validating more than the struggle, and using language that contextualizes difficulties and recognizes universality:

- *Validate more than hardship and struggle ("widen the lens").* It can be important when validating to include healthy aspects of experience that are being overshadowed by the difficulties present. For instance, if someone describes being defeated by setbacks, as well as validating this difficulty, we might bring into awareness and validate their hard work, in the group and at home—for example: "*It's great that you are still able to come to the group and support others, even after a night of terrible voices and very little sleep. I know we all appreciate your commitment to being here and supporting the group.*"

- *Validate using language that contextualizes the difficulty.* We seek to instill hope and motivation using language that locates or contextualizes specific difficulties in a particular time and place—for example: "*So, you were too scared to go out and meet your friend, and in that moment, it felt like it was too much to bear, that you couldn't carry on. That's how it felt sitting there on Saturday.*" While there is no challenge of the person's perspective or distress, contextualizing the difficulty in this way implicitly raises the possibility that this experience may not extend to all other times and situations.
- *Validate using language that recognizes universality.* As facilitators, we endeavor to use language that conveys how the person's experiences are both understandable and similar to what others have described—for example: "*How do others manage when feeling exhausted by a night of terrible voices or images and very little sleep?*" or "*Has anyone else been too scared to go out and meet friends or family, afraid that they'd be targeted if they did?*"

When offered in this way, validation can instill hope and support group cohesion (two key group factors in mindfulness for psychosis; see Chapter 6) and has the benefit of protecting group facilitators from becoming discouraged or weighed down by people's experience of the tyranny of psychosis.

Building Universality

People in mindfulness for psychosis groups consistently rate *universality*—the recognition that others have similar experiences—as the most important therapeutic group factor contributing to the process of change (see Chapter 6). Universality undermines the unhelpful metacognitive belief that "*I am fundamentally different and set apart from other people.*"

Feelings of universality are a powerful source of self-acceptance for people with psychosis. During each period of inquiry, facilitators seek one or two opportunities to highlight universality, by either (1) opening an individual's contribution to the group by asking if others have similar experiences—for example: "*I'm just wondering, has anyone else felt this fear when traveling on a bus or train?*" or (2) linking an individual's contribution to something that has previously been shared by another group member—for example: "*This reminds me of when Imran talked about having to get off the bus a mile from home because the fear of being attacked got too strong.*"

Guiding Discovery

Guided discovery is the main method facilitators use during inquiry to support metacognitive insights—the generalizable beliefs about internal experience that support people to transform their relationships with psychosis and themselves (see Chapter 2). Our approach to guided discovery owes much to the principles articulated by Padesky, who has written extensively on this in relation to cognitive-behavioral therapy (CBT) and psychotherapy more broadly (Padesky, 1993; Padesky & Kennerley, 2023). Guided discovery involves asking questions that draw a person's attention to potentially useful information outside their current awareness, listening carefully (and being open to hearing what's not expected), reflecting and summarizing to demonstrate and check understanding, and then asking analytical or synthesizing questions to elicit learning (Padesky & Kennerley, 2023).

A difference between guided discovery as used in CBT and in mindfulness for psychosis is that in CBT guided discovery is typically focused on unhelpful beliefs associated with distress or disability, and involves bringing these into awareness, reflecting on the beliefs and linked evidence, utility and impact, and developing alternatives. In mindfulness for psychosis, guided discovery focuses primarily on learning from moments of decentered awareness drawn from mindfulness practice or everyday life. Facilitators support the person to reflect on these experiences and explore "*What can we learn from this?*" to support metacognitive insights about psychosis, distress and well-being, or the self.

As when guiding discovery in CBT, facilitators:

- Embody an attitude of openness, curiosity, and a wish to learn together
- Ask questions and share reflections rather than telling people what to think
- Notice (and desist from) any urges to persuade people to think differently or *change minds*
- Ask analytical (e.g., "*What do you make of this?*") and synthesizing questions (e.g., "*How does this fit with the idea that you have no control over your life?*") rather than providing answers and solutions before the person has had time to reflect.

When discussing validation (see above), we introduced the importance of *widening the lens* to include experience that is likely to be useful but currently outside the person's awareness. This is an important feature of guided discovery, too. For example, imagine a person says after a mindfulness practice: "*I was lost the whole time. I couldn't even hear what you were saying. Mindfulness just isn't helping me. I just keep reacting the same as before to these thoughts and images.*" Three increasingly direct ways to bring overlooked experience into awareness are paradoxical injunction, direct questioning, and offering reminders:

- *Paradoxical injunction* reflects back what is said in a way that emphasizes the most extreme version of the point made—for example: "*So it's not helping at all, that's how it feels. There haven't been even a few brief moments during the practices when you have been able to step back. Is that right?*" Often this nudges people to recognize that there have been some such moments, albeit few and fleeting.
- *Asking directly* if there are any such moments can also help widen awareness—for example: "*So it feels as if nothing is changing. I wonder, have there been any moments during the practices over the last few weeks when you have been able to step back and pause before reacting? Even just for a few moments?*"
- *Gentle reminders* can draw people's attention to times that they may not have in mind at that moment—for example: "*Right, so today it really feels as if nothing is changing. [Pause] I'm just remembering what you shared last week, how last week you were able to step back and not react, and how that gave you some peace—do you remember that? I can see it's hard to keep this in mind today.*"

When guiding discovery, it can be useful for facilitators to ask ourselves: "*Is this person overlooking any potentially important experiences? What are they not able to connect with in this moment?*" Also, to reduce the likelihood of someone feeling criticized when widening the lens, we normalize this process and build universality by recognizing how (for all of us, facilitators too) our attention narrows when we are feeling low, threatened, or stressed.

In Chapter 2 we discussed how metacognitive insight involves new learning *about internal experience or the self*. When an individual in a group articulates a new metacognitive insight during inquiry, they are demonstrating new learning. For other group members, facilitators can make reflections and ask questions to explore whether this may also be relevant to them (supporting universality in the process)—for example:

"What do others think about this?" or *"Does this fit for anyone else?"* or *"Does what Imran said make sense for anyone else?"* When group members respond, we can follow this up to support people to articulate this learning in a way that fits for them—for example: "OK, *great, so this idea seems to make sense for you too, Izzy. Can you say more about how this fits with your experience of hearing voices?"*

Linking Guided Discovery to the Two-Circles Framework

The two-circles framework (see Chapter 2, Figure 2.1) describes common elements of distressing reaction and mindful responding to psychosis. As facilitators, we seek to use reflections, summaries, and questions to enable people to articulate metacognitive insights. This can be done by listening for examples of distressing reaction and mindful responding, bringing these clearly into awareness, and contrasting these two ways of relating to psychosis (see Figure 5.1).

Guided discovery is used to draw out the phenomenology of these different ways of relating to psychosis—how each feels in the mind, body, and emotionally (cf. Kabat-Zinn, 1994, 2013). Understanding derived from moments of mindful responding are then crystalized in the form of metacognitive insights—for example: *"When I react in these ways, I feel . . ."* and *"When I respond mindfully, I feel . . ."* Having drawn out the contrasting effects of distressing reaction and mindful responding, guided discovery then moves to the potential benefits of letting go of reactivity and choosing to respond mindfully to psychosis and other unpleasant sensations.

Linking Guided Discovery of Metacognitive Insights to the Core Process of Change

As a reminder, the two-circles framework describes distressing reaction and mindful responding to psychosis, and the core process of change describes how people move from distressing reaction to mindful responding. In any given moment, we do not have a target metacognitive insight in mind that we would like a person to come to. Each person in a group will discover and express metacognitive insights relevant to them, at

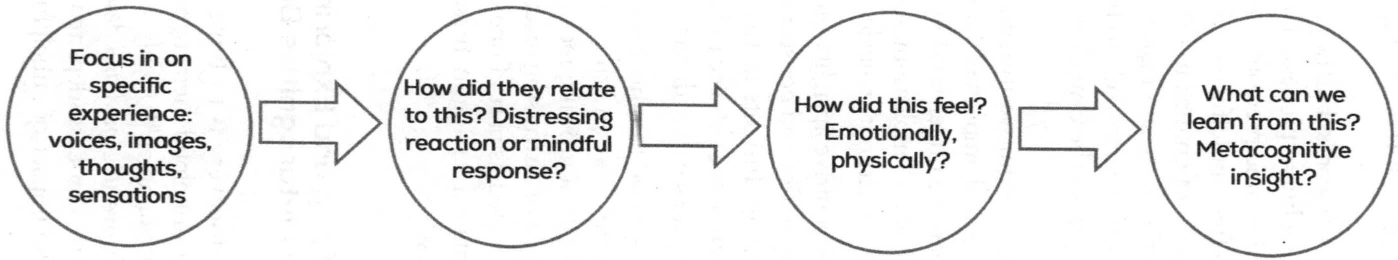

FIGURE 5.1. The process of guided discovery with unpleasant psychosis experiences.

their own pace, and in their own words. Furthermore, therapeutic learning is an iterative rather than a linear process. That said, time for group reflection and inquiry is a limited and precious commodity. To maximize opportunities for learning to free oneself from the tyranny of psychosis, facilitators keep the core process of change in mind (see Chapter 3, Figure 3.1), which helps frame reflections, summaries, and questions. In line with the core process of change, we are likely to hear different metacognitive insights at different points in the 8-week program:

- *Early sessions:* Early metacognitive insights often relate to recognizing the emotional and physical impact of habitual distressing reactions to psychosis, and an emerging understanding that sometimes it may be possible to step back and allow unpleasant sensations to come into awareness and then pass or fade without struggle.
- *Middle sessions:* Metacognitive insights often capture an understanding of the contrasting qualities and consequences of habitual reactions versus mindful responding. Insights at this stage in the program may express an emerging awareness of choice in how to relate to psychosis, and therefore personal influence over distress and well-being.
- *Later sessions:* Metacognitive insights toward the end of the program may describe how mindfulness can bring a sense of autonomy and control over the mind and body, a growing reclaiming of power. People start to recognize how, stripped of distressing reactivity, psychosis experiences deflate and can be accepted as part of one's life. This in turn may lead to metacognitive insights expressing increased self-acceptance and a sense of common humanity.

Identifying and Exploring Unhelpful Metacognitive Beliefs

A related focus for guided discovery is to bring clearly into awareness and reduce the influence of unhelpful metacognitive beliefs that maintain habitual reactivity—for example: "*It is only my struggle and resistance that stop me from being totally overwhelmed and destroyed*" (see Chapter 2, Table 2.1). Each iteration of this process (depicted in Figure 5.2) helps all group members recognize the impact of unhelpful metacognitive beliefs

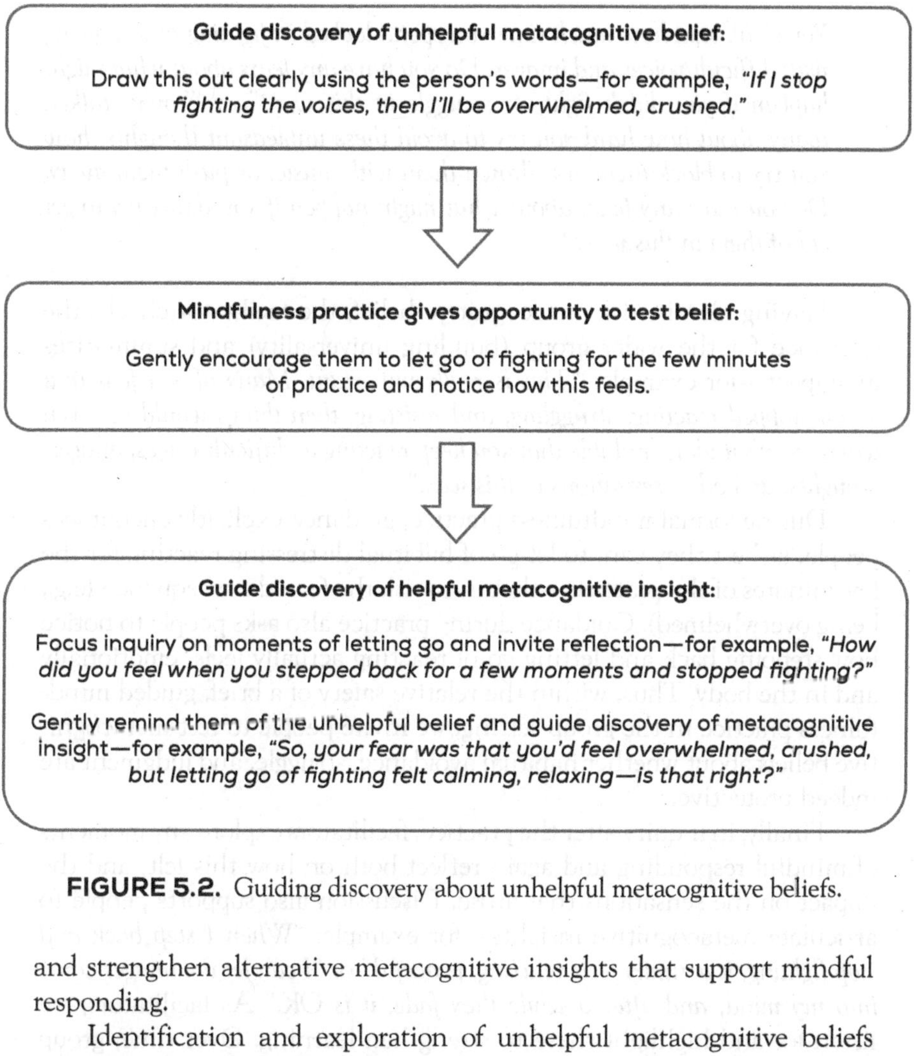

FIGURE 5.2. Guiding discovery about unhelpful metacognitive beliefs.

and strengthen alternative metacognitive insights that support mindful responding.

Identification and exploration of unhelpful metacognitive beliefs begins when facilitators draw out the impact of specific beliefs maintaining habitual reaction to unpleasant psychosis experience (avoiding, struggling, judging). Sometimes during group reflection, a person may simply state an unhelpful metacognitive belief, perhaps saying, *"I can't bear this,"* or *"The voices are too powerful—if I don't fight back, they'll crush me."* At other times, facilitators may need to draw these out, perhaps by exploring people's reactions and motivation for these, such as fears about stepping back and letting go of reacting. For example:

> *"You've all said how much time you spend locked in fighting or struggling with difficult voices and images. Do you have any fears about what might happen if you didn't fight, or struggle in this way?"* or *"You've talked today about how hard you try to avoid these unpleasant thoughts, how you try to block them out, drown them with music, or push them away. Do you have any fears about what might happen if you didn't try to get rid of them in this way?"*

Having identified a metacognitive belief, the facilitator checks the relevance for the wider group (building universality) and summarizes its impact—for example: *"This is really important. Many of you fear that if you stopped reacting, struggling, and resisting, then things would get even worse. So it's understandable that you keep reacting to difficult voices, images, thoughts, and other sensations in this way."*

During formal mindfulness practice, guidance explicitly encourages people, as best they can, to let go of habitual distressing reacting for the few minutes of the practice—that is, to risk the feared consequence (e.g., being overwhelmed). Guidance during practice also asks people to notice how stepping back and letting go of reacting actually feels, emotionally and in the body. Thus, within the relative safety of a brief, guided mindfulness practice in the group setting, we invite people to test metacognitive beliefs about whether habitual avoidance, struggle, and judgment are indeed protective.

Finally, in inquiry after the practice, facilitators explore any moments of mindful responding and again reflect both on how this felt, and the impact on the sensations that arose. Discussion also supports people to articulate metacognitive insights—for example: *"When I step back and stop fighting, it actually feels relaxing, peaceful"* or *"I can let the images come into my mind, and after a while they fade, it is OK."* As facilitators, we listen for and highlight these to strengthen learning. Over time, group members discover that while unhelpful metacognitive beliefs seem compelling, direct experience during mindfulness practice does not support them.

We recognize this is a lot to keep in mind. As facilitators, we do not need to get guided discovery *right* each time; we often return to missed opportunities later in the session, pick these up during the following session, or wait until they arise again.

6

Setting Up the Group and Facilitating Group Factors

A distinctive feature of mindfulness for psychosis groups is the explicit framing of the program as a therapeutic group rather than a skills class. The framing of a program matters because it sets the context for the focus and facilitation of the group—the change that might be possible, how we listen, and what we choose to attend to in sessions.

We frame mindfulness for psychosis groups in this way for three main reasons. First, the core process of change (see Chapter 3) is essentially a therapeutic process: Stepping back from self-defeating reactive mental habits, reclaiming one's power and agency, and self-acceptance are all cornerstones of psychotherapeutic change. Second, and linked to this, almost all people with psychosis who have come to our groups did so because of emotional distress, difficulty coping and living with psychosis, and a lack of self-acceptance. Framing the group as facilitating a therapeutic process therefore aligns with the experience and hopes of group members. A third reason is to foreground key group factors (Yalom, 1995), which contribute to the process of change in mindfulness for psychosis, and which facilitators actively attend to in order to maximize the therapeutic benefits of learning mindfulness for psychosis together.

In this chapter we offer guidance for facilitators on (1) the practicalities of setting up a group, and (2) how to support key group factors: universality, cohesion and belonging, hope, and being oneself more fully.

Practicalities of Setting Up a Group

How Many Facilitators?

We recommend two facilitators. During sessions, this gives group members two people to connect with and different perspectives on mindfulness. Additionally, having two facilitators makes it easier to cover the session content and to observe wider group processes. Following sessions (and during session breaks), co-facilitators are a source of mutual support, feedback, and learning. Sharing responsibility for running the group also reduces potential stress for facilitators.

Facilitators bring different, ideally complementary, expertise: one may have more experience of mindfulness, the other of working with people with psychosis. Co-facilitating with a person with lived experience of psychosis is an opportunity we have greatly valued. Differences in facilitators' age, sex, and ethnicity can add to the balance and diversity of a group. We also know that having two facilitators is not always possible. We have facilitated successful groups alone aided by an actively engaged supervisor.

How Many Group Members?

We recommend starting groups with 8–10 people with psychosis and not going above 12 members. When more than 10 group members are present, inquiry risks becoming either a quick check-in with everyone or missing out on some members, and opportunities are fewer for supporting metacognitive insight and deepening group factors. Having at least eight members protects against the group becoming unviable when some people do not attend or drop out, as it is still possible to facilitate rich inquiry, and build universality, cohesion, hope, and being oneself more fully, with just five or six people.

Is It Preferable to Recruit Based on Presenting Problems?

We are often asked if it is better to have groups where people all share a common psychosis experience, such as voices. This can provide an immediate basis for universality and cohesion. However, we have run mindfulness groups for people with shared and diverse presentations, and found that universality and cohesion build in both. For this reason, we neither recommend nor discourage single-presentation groups.

What is important is trying to avoid having one person with a different experience of psychosis from all other members (e.g., being the only person to have grandiose beliefs), as this can make it difficult for that person to develop a sense of universality and cohesion. In an ideal world, we would also seek to balance other important characteristics such as age, sex, and ethnicity. With small group numbers, this is not always possible, and we prioritize balancing psychosis experience and trust group members to value and respect individual differences.

Are There Any Exclusion Criteria?

Risk Assessment and Management of Harm

Facilitators new to mindfulness for psychosis groups are sometimes deterred by concerns about risk. In our experience, active risk behavior during a group is extremely rare. Furthermore, there is no evidence that contemporary mindfulness-based therapies are harmful for people with psychosis (O'Brien-Venus et al., 2024).

These groups were developed working in UK National Health Service (NHS) mental health services. People with psychosis in these services typically present with complex difficulties and needs, almost always including some risk (usually to themselves). One of us worked for many years in an inpatient ward and delivered mindfulness groups in this setting. We have also escorted people from and back to an inpatient ward to join a community group. We cannot recall a single instance of self-harm or attempted harm of another person during a mindfulness for psychosis group that we have facilitated.

Our intention is always to be as inclusive as possible, and this guiding principle has served us well. When potential group members are known to pose a particularly high risk, we hold individual pre-group meetings with them (see Chapter 7) and liaise with relevant staff to assess risk, triggers, and likely impact of attending the group. Decisions can then be made collaboratively with the person as to whether to join a mindfulness group immediately or wait for a future group.

Once a group is underway, it is important that facilitators apply the same approach to risk management as for any other group of people with mental health needs. Take whatever steps you would usually take in your setting. In our settings, our approach to risk management is always to know who to contact and what procedures to follow in the event of any active risk behaviors to self or others.

Use of Drugs and Alcohol

Many people use drugs and alcohol as ways of coping with psychosis—for example, to dampen the intensity of unpleasant voices, images, or sense of persecution, or their emotional responses to these. We do not exclude people from joining a mindfulness group on this basis and are tolerant of these choices between sessions, as long as this does not disrupt the group. We do ask people to commit to minimize using recreational drugs or alcohol prior to sessions, though we recognize this is not possible for everyone.

Medication Side Effects

Many people who have attended mindfulness groups are on high doses of psychiatric medication, which reduce concentration and energy. We would not exclude someone on this basis, as long as this does not disrupt the group. We may discuss with the prescribing professional the relative benefits of high doses of medication where side effects are interfering with an individual's ability to engage in the program.

Readiness to Change

Openness to learning mindfulness comes in part from fatigue and frustration with current ways of coping. When people remain committed to how they currently cope with and relate to psychosis sensations, our experience is that they are less likely to benefit from joining the program. This can be explored with individuals at a pre-group meeting. Even so, we do not exclude someone from joining a group for this reason—mindfulness can still be valuable as an additional way of relating to psychosis experience and supporting recovery, and group membership supports universality, empowerment, and self-acceptance.

Session Duration and Holding a Midsession Break

We recommend that sessions last 90 minutes with a 10- to 15-minute break. A break gives group members time to rest, take a comfort break and, if they wish, talk together. For facilitators, this gives time to reflect together and plan the second half of the session, check in with individuals if there are any concerns, and spend a few minutes connecting with group members.

The Physical Environment

It is important to attend to the physical environment when offering mindfulness for psychosis groups in person. We try to ensure everyone has clear access to the door—this fosters a sense of safety as people can see they can leave if they need to, and reduces any anxiety about disturbing others. We always sit in chairs for mindfulness practice. Try to make sure chairs are comfortable and spaced out, that the room is suitable, clean, uncluttered, and ideally has a window and pleasant view, which can help put people at ease. If you cannot access a pleasant space, then it can help to acknowledge the limitations of the venue you have, and explain that you wanted to offer the group now rather than delay while seeking a more suitable room.

The Benefits of Learning Mindfulness Together in a Group: Therapeutic Group Factors

Four interrelated group factors are particularly important contributors to engagement and change in mindfulness for psychosis groups: universality, group cohesion and belonging, instilling hope, and being myself more fully (cf. Yalom, 1995). The interrelatedness of these factors strengthens as the program progresses. The group factors reinforce one another and coalesce in a growing sense of autonomy, reclaiming power, and self-acceptance—the final stages of the core process of change in mindfulness for psychosis (see Chapter 3).

While group members usually start to experience these group factors from the earliest sessions, individuals inevitably have setbacks during the course of the program, and some may be temporarily thrown back into feeling unsafe, different, hopeless, and alone. As the group progresses, these setbacks are often shorter and less intense, and facilitators can explore differences in duration and intensity of setbacks as well as validating current difficulty and distress. Experiencing setbacks is a further source of universality, and having other group members acknowledge this often fosters group cohesion and belonging.

As interrelated factors, all four are likely to be operating in all eight sessions. With careful facilitation, each factor develops cumulatively over the course of the group, and generalizes into people's daily lives (see Table 6.1). As with the therapeutic processes represented in the core process of change, the development of group processes is not linear but iterative.

TABLE 6.1. Four Interrelated Group Factors Underpinning the Core Process of Change

Therapeutic group factor	How this presents and develops in mindfulness for psychosis groups
Universality	• Discovering others have similar experiences, problems, and hopes • Recognizing my capacity for connection, joy, and kindness • Discovering I am not different from other people
Group cohesion and belonging	• Sense of psychological safety and trust in the group • Feeling understood, supported, and accepted by the group • Believing I fit and belong here • Expressing kindness and altruism toward others
Hope	• Learning to "step back" from voices, images, thoughts, and other sensations, and that I do not always have to react • Feeling more in control of my mind and emotional health and well-being • Discovering I have more choice to live in line with what's important to me
Being myself more fully	• Breaking the silence—talking more openly about difficult voices, images, thoughts, feelings, and trauma • Sharing more of who I am, including moments of connection, joy, and kindness • Learning to be and trust myself

Universality

Universality—the discovery that others have similar experiences (Yalom, 1995)—has emerged as the single most important nonspecific group factor in mindfulness for psychosis groups (Chadwick et al., 2005, 2009). This is unsurprising. People with psychosis often feel set apart from others, sometimes to the point of seeing themselves as less than human. Self-dehumanization has a pervasive and corrosive impact. Many people fear that even in a group for people with psychosis, they will feel different, damaged, and alone. Discovering universality is therefore a powerfully humanizing process in these groups (O'Brien-Venus et al., 2023).

Universality typically begins with the discovery that others have similar experiences of psychosis, distress, and trauma. This is a vital first step, as it is often these experiences that drive emotionally laden beliefs about being different and set apart from others. Early in the group program, universality is also found in the shared daily struggle to cope and live with the impact of psychosis and trauma. From Session 2 onward, the practice of sharing moments of joy and connection in daily life extends opportunities for universality beyond problems and distress to times of joy and connection. Over time, universality becomes person based (as opposed to experience based), when people start to recognize the metacognitive insights that "*I am not different*" and "*I am a person like all others.*" This can be a profound shift in a person's sense of self, a far cry from initial feelings of being different, alone, and less than human. Over time, universality can also generalize to relationships outside the group when people recognize common experience with family, friends, and others.

Throughout the program, facilitators seek opportunities to build universality during guided practices, inquiry, psychoeducation, and other periods of discussion by (1) opening an individual's contribution to the group, exploring if others have similar experiences—for example: "*I'm just wondering, has anyone else felt this way when traveling on a bus or train?*" or (2) linking an individual's contribution to something that has been shared previously by another group member—for example: "*What you have shared reminds me of when Mo talked about having to get off the bus a mile from home because the fear and shame were so strong.*" In a group that feels safe, validating, and nonjudgmental, group members quickly begin to voice universality and facilitators need only use light-touch questions and comments linking people's experiences to create opportunities for universality to emerge.

Group Cohesion and Belonging

Group members will hear malevolent, omnipotent voices, see disturbing images, and experience paranoia and other difficult or confusing thoughts and feelings during mindfulness practices and inquiry. The beginnings of group cohesion lie in establishing a sense of psychological and physical safety in the group. Perceived physical safety is a real issue, as voices and paranoia can lead people to fear that they will be harmed in some way in the group (e.g., voices saying that facilitators will experiment on them, or harm them). Initial feelings of safety come from the containment of setting group agreements and from facilitators' unwavering validation, acceptance, and finding value in each person's contribution. As fears of being judged, rejected, or harmed ease, people's sense of threat reduces and is replaced by a growing recognition that they are understood, supported, and accepted by the group. This develops into a sense of group cohesion and belonging, and we have heard people in several groups talk of "*the mindfulness group*" as a valued shared identity. This process can happen quite quickly or take several sessions, especially if people are thrown back into a state of threat by difficult life events.

Over time, the sense of trust and belonging often begins to generalize to relationships outside the group. This can empower people to engage with new opportunities in daily life, in line with what is most important to them. Facilitators pay increased attention to these steps toward personal recovery as the program progresses, and particularly in Sessions 7 and 8 (see Chapter 12).

Instillation of Hope

Hope builds through emerging universality and cohesion, as well as people learning that they can engage in moments of mindfulness. As they learn to step back and let go of habitual reactions to unpleasant sensations, group members feel increasingly empowered and the sense of being overwhelmed by psychosis diminishes. People describe being more in control in relation to their psychosis, and having more choice in their lives. Sharing moments of joy and connection at the start of each group also instills hope for more of these experiences in the future.

The growing sense of hope strengthens feelings of power and control, and engenders personal autonomy. Like the other group factors, we seek to support people to generalize increased hope and autonomy beyond the group. This typically leads to people making changes in their daily lives, which in turn strengthens hopes for personal recovery, and expectations that they can do the things that are important to them, and live well with psychosis.

Being Myself More Fully

Many people will have avoided talking about psychosis and any past trauma, even with family and friends, given fears of being judged and rejected, and shame associated with stigma (Skrobinska et al., 2024). An important step toward self-acceptance is to break this silence—to dare to name psychosis and any trauma in the group. It is important that facilitators manage this carefully, supporting people to name these experiences safely, without going into detail that would be better shared in individual therapy, and attending to the impact on others in the group.

Another way in which people can express and be themselves more fully is to share moments of joy and connection. It is important that facilitators recognize that this too can feel exposing—for people to dare to reveal aspects of their wider lives and selves. With effective facilitation, this can lead to recognizing a shared human capacity for joy and connection, and the metacognitive insight that "*I am more than the psychosis.*"

Having these experiences heard, validated, and accepted by facilitators and other group members increases people's willingness to express and be themselves more fully, and this is a significant step toward self-acceptance. Facilitators' willingness to share some of their own limitations and fallibility models how *being myself more fully* involves vulnerability, not perfection.

Facilitator Attitudes That Support Therapeutic Factors

Facilitators seek to support the therapeutic group factors by embodying three foundational attitudinal qualities: authenticity, acceptance, and trust (see Figure 6.1). These attitudes and linked behaviors have guided

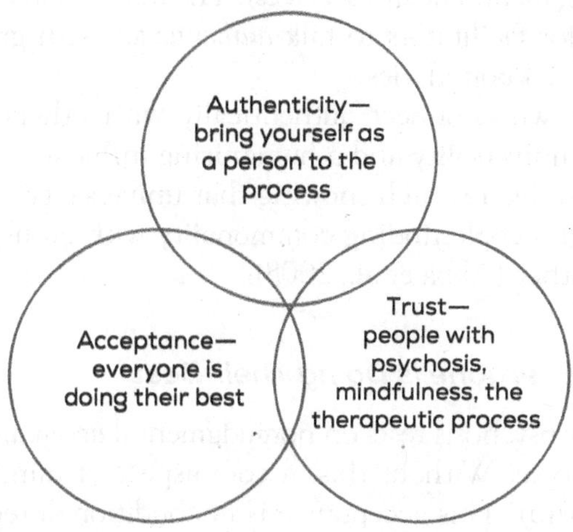
Authenticity—
bring yourself as
a person to the
process
Acceptance—
everyone is
doing their best
Trust—
people with
psychosis,
mindfulness, the
therapeutic process

FIGURE 6.1. Facilitator attitudes that support group factors.

us well, and we recommend facilitators lean into these in moments of uncertainty or difficulty in sessions.

Authenticity: Facilitators Being Themselves More Fully

In mindfulness for psychosis groups, we recognize that everyone brings expertise. Group members are experts by experience, and many bring additional relevant expertise—for example, having attended a previous group. Facilitators bring their professional expertise and may also have relevant lived experience.

Alongside their professional expertise, *facilitators need to bring themselves as people to the process.* Our aspiration to *meet the person not the problem* requires that we too be ourselves. This is central to the art of facilitating groups and we encourage facilitators to explore this in supervision.

In this way, running a mindfulness for psychosis group is an opportunity for facilitators, alongside group members, to explore being themselves more fully. This includes judicial self-disclosure—that is, disclosure that is likely to benefit group members given the aims and focus of the group. For example, it is normalizing and encouraging for group members to hear how facilitators also get lost in reactivity, which helps dispel the myth that there are people without problems (group facilitators and other professionals) and people with problems (group members and others using mental health services). The midsession break also gives a few minutes for facilitators to talk *authentically* with group members, within professional boundaries.

Facilitators who connect authentically with others in the group are a source of universality and a humanizing influence. This is consistent with qualitative research showing that universality in these groups emerges through people finding commonality with group facilitators as well as one another (Abba et al., 2008).

Acceptance: Everyone Is Doing Their Best

Mindfulness for psychosis rests on nonjudgmental *acceptance* of all group members as people. Without this, a core aspect of mindfulness is lost (Kabat-Zinn, 2013). This acceptance is unconditional, regardless of the person's history, behavior, or progress, and includes their right to choose the direction in which they change (Rogers, 1961).

Facilitators model acceptance through consistently warm, validating, and balanced speech and body language. It is always possible to find something to value and validate in each person's contributions. If someone arrives late, we may thank them for attending and supporting others. If someone has not practiced all week, we may appreciate their practice in the session. Balance in speech also means not being overly enthusiastic when someone reports significant progress, as this can then make it hard not to seem less supportive if the next person describes how they aren't finding mindfulness helpful. We seek to bring the same warmth and validation to everyone.

Embodying acceptance is especially important when difficulties arise. Facilitators keep in mind how each person is doing their best in their present circumstances. Mindfulness is historically rooted in an understanding that, for us all, our *best* will change moment-to-moment according to a vast matrix of ever-changing conditions (Rahula, 1959). Facilitators can return with genuine curiosity to the question, *What can we learn from what is happening right now?* to guide tricky moments during mindfulness groups.

To truly embody acceptance is "*by no means an easy thing*" (Rogers, 1961, p. 20). As facilitators, we do the best we can throughout the 8-week program, while stepping back from seeking perfection. Acceptance is an aspiration and practice, not a demand, and invites personal acceptance that this will be imperfect. We find it helps us establish a nonjudgmental group culture if we keep in mind, and potentially express, our belief that everyone is doing their best to engage with mindfulness and the group, and how, for all of us, our best—that is, what is possible—will change from one moment to another.

Trust

We seek to *trust* people with psychosis, mindfulness, and the therapeutic process:

> People often have said to me over the years that to offer mindfulness for psychosis takes courage. I see it differently. What empowers me is trust; trust in people with psychosis individually and in a group, trust in mindfulness, and trust in the core humanising therapeutic process. To truly offer mindfulness for psychosis in any moment requires that we free ourselves from fear and prejudice and reach out to the

> person; and that we trust in the person's capacity to connect with us in this way, and to make choices for themselves about what is possible. (Chadwick, 2019, p. 319)

To be trusted is empowering for group members, and empowerment is essential for recovery. Even when people may be lacking hope and trust in themselves, we want to convey our hope and expectation for their recovery, and our confidence that they will be able to find a way to live well with psychosis. We also need to trust that mindfulness can benefit people with psychosis through the core therapeutic process. Keeping this in mind frees facilitators from feeling personally responsible for participants' engagement and recovery in ways that are unhelpful (see Chapter 13).

Addressing Behaviors That Threaten Group Functioning

It is rare for participants to behave in ways that threaten group functioning. If such behaviors do arise (e.g., behaving unkindly or disrespectfully to others), this both breaks group agreements and weakens the group factor of cohesion and belonging. Facilitators first seek gently and collaboratively to reaffirm the breached group agreements and then to focus on reestablishing cohesion for all in the group. We may also decide to meet individually with those involved after the session to check that any issues have been resolved. Generally, we have found that people with psychosis are very understanding and forgiving of others' struggles and occasional behavioral lapses.

We have never encountered physical violence in a mindfulness for psychosis group. If someone were to present a risk to themselves or others, facilitators should follow their relevant service protocols, prioritizing the physical safety of all present. This is likely to involve calling for support and ending the group session.

When people experience a setback in relation to group cohesion, it is important that facilitators return to the primary task of establishing a sense of psychological and physical safety as the foundation for developing cohesion and belonging in the group. Behaviors that threaten group cohesion include attending under the influence of substances, dominating discussions or remaining silent, and a lack of interest in learning mindfulness.

Attending Sessions under the Excessive Influence of Recreational Drugs or Alcohol

If we suspect this to be the case, rather than raising it in front of the group, we would without judgment talk with the person individually at the next opportunity, typically after the session or during the midsession break (when we could decide together whether they stay for the second half). We stress the importance of keeping use of drugs and alcohol to a minimum during the group program, and explain that if the person were to attend again under the influence of excessive drugs or alcohol, we would need to ask them not to return. We would discuss alternative sources of help, including dedicated drug and alcohol services if this was a primary problem. The aim is to reach a compassionate and collaborative decision that works for both the individual and the group. People are warmly encouraged to join a future group where appropriate.

Dominating Discussions

If someone repeatedly speaks too much, or interrupts others, facilitators first use subtle verbal and nonverbal cues to try to shape their behavior, such as turning toward another person and inviting them to contribute. If this was unsuccessful, they would address the person directly—for example: *"John, can I just stop you there? What you've shared about living with paranoia is important. Let's see if others have similar experience."* Occasionally even this more direct approach does not work, and we need to meet with the person individually to ask for their help in creating more space for others to speak, framed both as an altruistic action and an opportunity to hear and learn from others.

Remaining Silent

Sometimes in a session, one or two people may say little or nothing, and yet remain attentive and engaged, which is fine. When an individual is persistently silent and they seem disconnected from the group, this can be unsettling for others, and so facilitators try to engage them more fully.

This can be as simple as making regular eye contact and offering a warm and encouraging smile. If the silence persists, facilitators can gently create opportunities for the person to speak during inquiry—for example: "*So, several people are beginning to really get a sense of what it means to step back from difficult thoughts and voices. May, how was the practice for you today?*" If the behavior still persists, we would meet with the person individually to seek to understand this and help them connect with the group in ways that feel manageable for them.

Lack of Interest in Learning Mindfulness

Occasionally, someone attends a group but seems to have little interest in practicing or discussing mindfulness. It may be that they are more focused on discussing their experience of psychosis more broadly, or past trauma, or concerns about mental health care received. Once again, we would suggest an individual meeting to remind them of the purpose of the group and consider whether alternative interventions (such as a voices group, individual therapy, or access to service feedback systems) might be a better fit.

In summary, behaviors that threaten group functioning are rare, and most can be anticipated and addressed at a pre-group meeting. On occasion, facilitators need to speak individually with group members to understand and jointly resolve issues. Group work is a rich opportunity not only for individuals to benefit in terms of therapeutic progress but to be able to express understanding and kindness toward others who may be struggling in this setting.

III

Mindfulness for Psychosis Groups

THE 8-WEEK PROGRAM

7

Holding an Optional Pre-Program Meeting

It can be useful to hold individual meetings with potential group members, particularly for novice facilitators. This provides an opportunity for people to meet one of the facilitators, hear about the aims and structure of the program, and raise any questions or concerns. A pre-group meeting can instill hope that the group may be useful, ease worries about participation, and so increase subsequent attendance. The aim is to support people to make a reasonably informed decision about whether to join a mindfulness for psychosis group.

Pre-group meetings allow us to (1) hear about the person's current experience of psychosis, including habitual distressing reactions; (2) guide a brief mindfulness practice; (3) describe the group aims, structure, and process; (4) hear and address any concerns about mindfulness for psychosis groups; and (5) support the person in deciding whether to join the coming group.[1]

This is not the time to complete a comprehensive psychological assessment. We do not seek a detailed understanding of the person's experience of psychosis, personal history, or unhelpful metacognitive beliefs. In a pre-group meeting we seek a broad-brush picture of their current relationship with psychosis, their openness to change, and whether joining a mindfulness group could be useful.

---

[1] In some settings it can be helpful to advertise an upcoming group—an example of a flyer or poster is given at *www.guilford.com/chadwick-materials*.

We usually address any concerns about mindfulness groups (Point 4 above) after hearing about the person's current relationship with psychosis, practicing mindfulness, and outlining the group aims and structure (Points 1–3 above). This is because the first three points often have the effect of easing fears and concerns about the program and being in a group. The simple way in which mindfulness is introduced and practiced in a pre-group meeting can reduce any worries about not being able to *do mindfulness* or this being a religious practice in this context. This sequence usually works well but it is a guide and it is important to be flexible and responsive to people's priorities. If someone starts a pre-group meeting with a strong concern about mindfulness—for example as being a form of mind control, then we would address this first and directly.

Holding a pre-group meeting is not essential, and we recognize that this is not always possible in busy service settings. We have led many successful groups where pre-group meetings were not held or only with some group members. That said, we strongly encourage novice facilitators to plan pre-group meetings, as this can be an effective way of engaging people who may understandably have mixed feelings about joining a mindfulness group, and is an opportunity to become familiar with elements of the program prior to leading a group.

Meet the Person, Not the Problem

At a pre-group meeting, the person with psychosis gains a first impression of how you relate to them and how it might feel to be part of a group that you lead. It is therefore important that you *meet the person, not the problem* (Chadwick, 2006). This might mean spending a few moments at the beginning of the meeting connecting with them and prioritizing their comfort and ease before focusing on the business or content of the meeting. For example:

FACILITATOR: It's good to meet you, Monica. How did you feel about coming along today?

MONICA: I felt a bit on edge. Last night and today the voices were strong, telling me to stay home where it's safe. I don't like going out, meeting new people [pause] but it was OK. I wanted to come as well.

FACILITATOR: So, it was tough getting here, having to travel, and meet me. The voices and fears were strong. Lots of people feel on edge before this kind of meeting; it's a very natural, very human way to feel. I can also see that part of you wanted to come along and find out more, which is great. So, well done! I'm glad you made it.

Even an individual pre-group meeting offers opportunities to foster the four group factors that support learning to respond mindfully to psychosis—universality, cohesion and belonging, hope, and being oneself more fully (see Chapter 6). We keep these group factors in mind from this first meeting and seek to communicate these implicitly through our verbal and nonverbal behaviors. It is important that this is done in a way that aligns with the facilitator qualities that support these group processes: authenticity, acceptance, and trust. We have observed novice therapists trying hard to communicate *genuine regard*, verbally and nonverbally, in ways that are well-intentioned but performative. Our experience is that people with psychosis recognize and can feel further alienated by such inauthenticity. Facilitators who prioritize authenticity are most able to put people at their ease, and are most effective in fostering the key group factors in mindfulness for psychosis groups.

We also want to communicate our confidence that people can learn to respond mindfully to psychosis, if they so choose. At a pre-group meeting, even when a person is describing highly distressing and traumatic experiences, we convey trust in them when we ask them if they are willing to try a 5-minute mindfulness practice with us, when we ask them to let us know if the practice becomes too difficult to stay with, and when we close our eyes and complete the practice together.

The Person's Current Experience of Psychosis

Exploration of the person's current experience of psychosis is present focused and covers three main points: (1) What are their *current* difficult psychosis experiences (voices, images, thoughts, etc.)?, (2) What are their usual ways of coping with these experiences?, and (3) What are some subjective advantages and disadvantages of these ways of coping?

The two-circles model (see Chapter 2, Figure 2.1) guides our exploration of the person's ways of coping, though we would not share it explicitly at this early stage. We look for examples of avoidance, struggle (rumination, worry, and confrontation), and judgment—that is, familiar distressing reactions on the left-hand side of the model. Using the person's own language, we might ask:

- *"How do you usually react when you hear the voices?"*
- *"How do you usually react when you have that feeling of being watched?"*
- *"How do you usually react when you see these 'horrible' images in your head?"*

Usually, a person will describe one or more distressing reactions depicted in the model. Discussions are always collaborative, a back-and-forth process of discovery, and when people are not able to put their ways of reacting into words, it can be helpful tentatively to inquire about specific reactions. For example:

- *"I wonder, do you ever try to avoid the voices, maybe try to distract yourself or block them out?"*
- *"Do you ever find yourself resisting or fighting the voices?"*
- *"When you have that feeling of being watched, do you ever find yourself going over and over things in your mind, trying to work it all out?"*
- *"I wonder, do you ever get caught up judging yourself as a person for having these 'horrible' images in your head?"*

The aim here is to identify examples of the main ways in which the person is reacting prior to introducing mindfulness as an alternative. We are not seeking a comprehensive assessment of all the person's coping strategies.

Next, we explore what the person sees as the advantages and disadvantages of their current ways of coping. How well do these work for the person, and what are the costs of continually reacting in these ways? Table 7.1 lists some common advantages and disadvantages that people describe.

Readiness to Change

When people are committed to how they *currently* cope with unpleasant psychosis sensations, our experience is that they are less likely to engage with mindfulness. At a pre-group meeting, we gauge whether the person

TABLE 7.1. Common Advantages and Disadvantages of Current Reactions to Psychosis, as Described by People Attending Mindfulness for Psychosis Groups

	Possible advantages	Disadvantages
Avoidance	• Short-term respite • Gives me a temporary sense of control	• Exhausting—drains time and energy • Often doesn't work or only for a short time • They (psychosis sensations) come back—stronger or at a worse time • Reinforces how powerful they seem
Struggle—rumination, worry, confrontation	• Feel like I'm prepared for danger • Doing something to find a way out, seek a solution	• Distressing and exhausting • Uses up so much of my time • Fuels hopelessness—I don't really get anywhere • Leaves me feeling defeated, powerless
Judging psychosis and myself	• Shows I don't agree with what they (the voices, persecutors, others) are saying	• Draining and distressing • Erodes my self-confidence • Drives self-hatred

is seeking a different relationship with psychosis and is open to mindfulness as a possible alternative.

Openness to mindfulness comes in part from a recognition of the costs and limitations of current coping, and a willingness to explore whether there might be an alternative to the endless cycle of avoidance, struggle, and judgment. In the rare instances when a person seems committed to maintaining their current relationship with psychosis, it can be helpful to explore their openness to change directly—for example: "*It sounds as if your current ways of managing the difficult voices and images are working quite well for you. Mindfulness does involve trying a different way of relating to voices and images. How do you feel about this?*"

Accepting Psychosis

We do not use the term *acceptance* or the concept of *accepting psychosis* at a pre-group meeting (or indeed in the early sessions of the program).

This is because this language can all too easily feel invalidating or be misunderstood as meaning resignation or agreement with the content of voices or thoughts (or the meaning ascribed to them; e.g., "*I'm worthless*"). The exception would be if a person introduces the term, then we would use this carefully to mean accepting that these experiences are happening right now.

Introducing Mindfulness as a New Way of Relating to Psychosis

Discussion of current ways of coping with psychosis forms the basis for introducing mindfulness as an alternative way of relating to difficult voices, images, thoughts, and other psychosis sensations. People's habitual reactions usually involve either attempts to block out and avoid psychosis sensations, or becoming caught up and lost in reactivity. We then introduce mindfulness as an alternative to both, For example:

> *"You've described how you either try to avoid the voices and thoughts or you end up locked in struggling with them. Neither is really working for you—you're worn out, and it's getting harder and harder to keep going. Mindfulness is a different way to relate to difficult voices and thoughts. We see if it's sometimes possible to take a middle way—to step back and let the voices and thoughts come and go without having to react to them, without getting stuck in either avoidance or struggle."*

Most people gather a broad understanding of mindfulness when introduced in this way, even if they doubt that they will be able to put this into practice, or that it will be helpful to them. To lessen any anxiety about changing their relationship with psychosis, we do not ask people to abandon current hard-won ways of coping. Instead, mindfulness is introduced as an additional way of coping. For example:

> *"You'll still have your other ways of coping. If you are having a tough day and you just need to sleep and zone out, that's OK. Mindfulness gives us some choice—we can choose how to respond in a situation, when to react, and when to step back and let things pass. In this way, learning mindfulness can give you some more control and choice."*

Introducing a Brief Mindfulness Practice

After asking about the person's current experience of psychosis and their usual ways of coping, and introducing mindfulness as a possible alternative, we suggest a brief mindfulness practice—for example: "*It's difficult to really understand what mindfulness is without doing it. Do you feel OK to practice together now, just for a few minutes? I'll guide us through it and then we can talk about how it went.*"

At the pre-group meeting we use a shortened (approximately 5-minute) version of the core mindfulness practice that we presented in Chapter 3. The shortened script is given in Appendix 7.1 at the end of this chapter (and you can find an audio recording of it at *www.guilford.com/chadwick-materials*). After this practice, we calmly congratulate the person, and then have a brief discussion—for example: "*The first thing to say is 'well done!' It's not easy to practice for the first time, it can feel scary or odd, but you did it. How was that for you?*"

The focus of inquiry at a pre-group meeting is threefold: (1) to begin to build a sense that mindfulness is doable (i.e., instill hope), perhaps lightly exploring if there were any moments of noticing bodily sensations, or breathing, or voices, images, and thoughts arising; (2) to look out for major misunderstandings about mindfulness (e.g., that it is supposed to create an empty mind); and (3) to show (and model) acceptance that the person is doing the best they can, always finding something encouraging to comment on—for example: If the practice was really tough and the person felt very scattered, we might say, "*So it was really tough, but you got through it,*" or "*It's great that there were a couple of moments of feeling connected to your breathing; we can build on that.*"

Introducing the Group Aims, Structure, and Process

We have found it is helpful to have a brief introduction to the aims of the group, and what this will look like in practice. Like all the psychoeducation elements of the sessions, this is brief. For example:

> "*Mindfulness for psychosis groups have been running for over 20 years and have helped many, many people. Mindfulness doesn't stop difficult voices, images, or thoughts from happening, but it can help people learn*

to live with them without feeling overwhelmed or dominated, without feeling that difficult voices, images, thoughts, and fears rule their lives."

Occasionally someone expresses disappointment that mindfulness won't get rid of their psychosis. When this happens, we validate how hard it is to live with these experiences and come back to the earlier discussion about how much distress and exhaustion come from being trapped in reaction—being lost in seemingly endless cycles of avoidance, struggle, and judgment—and how mindfulness can help with this.

Addressing Any Concerns about Attending a Mindfulness for Psychosis Group

It is important at the pre-group meeting to ask if the person has any concerns about joining the group. While we do not expect to ameliorate all concerns, we are demonstrating a willingness to hear and discuss doubts, fears, and worries as they arise. This willingness itself usually leaves people feeling less anxious, hopeless, or ashamed, and may increase subsequent group attendance.

We might simply say: *"Often when we think about joining a new group, or trying something new, we can feel some doubt or fear. Do you have any worries about joining a mindfulness group?"* Most people share one or more concerns related to four sources: mindfulness, personal ability and resilience, being in a group, and how change will impact the psychosis. Table 7.2 gives examples of specific concerns raised and possible responses. At this point, the aim is to hear and validate any such concerns, share how common these are, and highlight how these begin to ease quite quickly once the group is underway for most people. We do not inquire about all four domains in turn but respond to whichever are raised.

Reaching a Collaborative Decision about Joining a Mindfulness for Psychosis Group

Our stance when offering mindfulness for psychosis groups both in community and inpatient settings is to be as inclusive as possible. The pre-group meeting is not used as an assessment to select some and screen

TABLE 7.2. Common Concerns That Arise at Pre-Group Meetings, and Possible Responses

Source of concern	Concern	Possible responses (normalize, then reflect as follows)
Mindfulness	• It won't help me. • It'll make me worse. • Mindfulness is a religious thing, and I won't feel comfortable with it.	• Most people get some benefit from being in a mindfulness group. • The evidence is that it doesn't make people worse or harm them. • Mindfulness is about learning to notice what is happening, step back, and choose how we react—it helps us have more choice and control in our lives (there's nothing religious in what we do in these groups).
Me	• I won't be able to do it. • I can't concentrate. • It'll be too difficult and I'll fail. • I'm too unwell, my psychosis is too strong.	• It's about doing the best we can. • Whatever you manage to do is fine—there's no judgment and no failure. • We can all be a little more mindful in our lives and a little kinder to ourselves. • People with years of really strong voices, images, and paranoia have found the group helpful.
Being in a group	• I'll be different and will still be alone. • People will judge me. • I'll feel threatened by others. • It'll be too stressful.	• Many, many people feel different and alone—this group may help with that. • People in the group support and encourage each other, without judgment. • We will do all we can to ensure that the group feels safe for everyone. • It can be good talking to others with similar experiences, see you're not alone.
Impact on voices, images, perceived persecutors	• The voices and persecution will get worse, and I won't be able to cope. • It's too risky to change how I relate to psychosis.	• Voices and images do sometimes get a little worse for a while—this can happen anyway, and if it happens, you'll have the support of the group. • I think you are stronger than you realize. • Mindfulness helps people reclaim their power, choose how they relate to psychosis, and feel more in control of their lives—I hope you'll give this a try.

others out according to strict inclusion and exclusion criteria. Aside from very rare instances, where group attendance was deemed to bring an unmanageable risk of harm to the person or others in the group, we have not refused a person a place in a mindfulness group.

A key reason for leaning into such an inclusive approach is that we have found people with psychosis to be incredibly generous in their ability to accept one another in these groups. People show understanding and acceptance when a group member is caught up with paranoia, voices, or confusion, or if someone gets up and leaves partway through a session. This level of acceptance and tolerance often comes from shared experience; people have commented that *"I've been there," "I've had times when I've felt this way,"* or *"It's really tough, but it does pass."*

At the end of the pre-group meeting, the person is invited to consider whether they would like to join the group. The task for the person is to reach the best decision they can, informed by the initial mindfulness practice and collaborative discussion. For example:

> "Mo, *today we've talked through what it's been like living with psychosis. We've practiced mindfulness together and talked a little about how the groups run and what mindfulness might offer. How are you feeling about joining a group? Does this seem like the right thing for you now?"*

People with psychosis often feel as if they are living on a knife's edge. The combination of seemingly powerful, unpleasant psychosis sensations, and unhelpful metacognitive beliefs about the consequences of changing habitual ways of reacting, may lead people to decline to join a mindfulness group. We accept and support this. For example, Simon, a 19-year-old young man, heard a malevolent, omnipotent voice that commanded him to hurt other people, and either cut or kill himself. He believed the voice to be a devil. Every day he exhausted himself fighting with the voice, resisting the commands with all his might. He believed it was only his resistance that saved him from being overwhelmed and doing as the voice said. The idea of letting go of this fight was *"a mad idea"*—as if we were suggesting he let the devil overpower him and harm his family. Sometimes, people who decline mindfulness groups come back months or even years later. Respecting their decision and letting them know they can ask to be referred again in the future allows this to remain a possibility. Simon instead chose CBT to work on the voice omnipotence and his sense of self.

Sometimes, people are seeking an alternative approach. Perhaps the person is looking for more of a talking therapy, peer support, or employment advice. It is important to be familiar with local services so we can signpost or facilitate onward referrals where requested and indicated. As an example, Joe, a man in his 30s, had not worked for several years following a severe and prolonged episode of acute psychosis. Joe decided that he did not need to join a mindfulness group but would like some help getting back into work, so we arranged a meeting with a mental health vocational advisor.

Occasionally, we may be unsure whether mindfulness is likely to be beneficial. As discussed earlier, some people appear committed to current ways of coping, and others are hoping for a new medication or other medical intervention to *get rid of* their experiences. In these instances, we gently outline our approach and encourage the person to make a decision that is right for them at this time. We would not usually exclude them from a mindfulness group (unless unable to manage risk in this setting)—the evidence is that the program does not cause harm, and most people gain something, even if this comes more from therapeutic factors such as universality and belonging rather than learning mindfulness.

Where we see a good fit, we offer gentle and authentic encouragement. For example:

> *"Mindfulness has helped me a lot in my life, and I know mindfulness has helped many people with psychosis. From our discussion today I think you might find the group helpful and others could benefit from your contributions—give this some thought and let me know if you'd like to join the group."*

Finally, when a person agrees to join a mindfulness group, it can help to anticipate possible after-effects, just lightly. For example:

> *"Great, I'm glad you've decided to give it a go. Just to say, some people find they can feel a bit worried before their group starts, or maybe their voices suggest they don't come. If this happens, I hope you're able to come anyway. People settle into the group pretty quickly. We can all feel a little anxious before trying something new."*

APPENDIX 7.1. Brief Version of the Core Mindfulness Practice

Opening Phase

1. Let's start by taking a moment to sit comfortably in the chair, sitting in an upright, relaxed position with your feet resting on the floor. If it feels comfortable, allowing your eyes to close, or if you'd prefer, resting your gaze on the floor in front of you. It is easy to get locked in our mind, lost in thinking, so we begin mindfulness by bringing our awareness to our bodies. Gently bring your awareness to the soles of your feet on the floor. Really connect with the sensations in this place in your body—maybe noticing feelings of temperature, pressure. Now gently bringing your awareness up into your legs, your upper body, your head and face. Just noticing whatever sensations are present right now in your body, maybe noticing the pressure of the chair, or the feeling of clothing against your skin.

2. Now bring your awareness gently to the sensations in your body as you breathe in and as you breathe out. This might be noticing the rise and fall of your tummy or chest as you breathe in and out, or the tips of your nostrils, as the cooler air comes in and the slightly warmer air comes out.

Middle Phase

3. Our awareness moves naturally to other things—sounds, thoughts, voices, images, worries. As best we can, allowing each of these sensations to come into awareness, and then pass or fade into the background. Then gently returning to the breath.

4. Noticing when we get lost, maybe struggling with voices, caught up in worries or trying to work things out. We all get lost like this. As best you can, letting go of this struggle and reconnecting with the sensations of breathing—breathing in and out.

Closing Phase

5. For the last few seconds, really being open to whatever sensations arise, allowing these to come fully into awareness and then pass or fade without reacting. Then coming back to the sensations of breathing in and out.

6. When you are ready, gently open your eyes and settle back into the room.

From *Mindfulness for Psychosis: A Group Therapy Approach*, by Paul Chadwick, Katherine Newman-Taylor, and Nicola Abba. Copyright © 2027 The Guilford Press. Permission to photocopy this material, or to download and print enlarged versions (*www.guilford.com/chadwick-materials*), is granted to purchasers of this book for personal use or use with clients; see copyright page for details.

8

Overview of the Group Manual

The mindfulness for psychosis group manual emerged over many iterations of the program. The manual aligns with the two key theoretical frameworks and facilitator guidance described in this book. If you have not yet read these chapters, please do so first. This will support you in facilitating the program and moment-to-moment decision making during sessions, based on the principles and theory underpinning the approach rather than viewing the program as a series of sessional tasks.

The manual is not a tightly controlled and timed series of tasks for facilitators to complete. Nor is it intended to be used to push or drive forward a predetermined process of change, having everyone arrive at the same end point by Session 8. To use the manual in these ways would be to lose the essence of mindfulness.

Mindfulness for psychosis is a principle-led process. Effective facilitation of the program depends on using the session-by-session guidance flexibly, being willing to adjust your plans in response to group members' progress and needs. Content and guidance notes reflect the stage of learning where we have found most people to be at this point in the program. The process of change is iterative rather than linear, and individuals and whole groups can move at a different pace. As facilitators, we need to read the group—sometimes slow down a little, sometimes speed up a little.

The manual presents the eight sessions in four pairs: Sessions 1 and 2, 3 and 4, 5 and 6, and 7 and 8. Sessions are paired to align with the stages in the core process of change (see Chapter 3) while supporting flexibility in facilitation and acknowledging a degree of variability in how the process of change unfolds. It is unhelpful to try to pin down the emergence of, say, particular challenges or metacognitive insights to one specific session.

Session Theme and Structure

Each pair of linked sessions has an overarching theme describing a shared focus. Themes inform the psychoeducation, inquiry, and handouts for these sessions, and locate each session within an unfolding process of change. Each session runs for 90 minutes, with a 10- to 15-minute break, and follows the same simple structure:

1. Opening the session
2. Review mindfulness practice over the week
3. First core mindfulness practice
4. Inquiry focused on first practice
5. Psychoeducation—brief presentation of topic and linked reflective discussion

   [Optional break]

6. Second core mindfulness practice
7. Inquiry focused on second practice and session learning points
8. Closing the session and home practice

A consistent session structure helps group members and facilitators know what is coming, stay on track in sessions, and be flexible (e.g., adjusting psychoeducational material across adjacent sessions for a group moving at a different pace from that suggested here).

Opening the Session and Reviewing Mindfulness Practice over the Week

Facilitators open sessions with a warm welcome and reminder of the session number. We may tune people into the session by acknowledging that simply getting here takes real commitment, highlighting that people's attendance supports others as well as themselves, or mentioning a key learning point from the previous session.

From Session 2 onward, facilitators check in on formal practice and informal moments of mindfulness (e.g., stepping back and not reacting to a provoking comment from a family member). For both formal and informal mindfulness practice, we are interested in how this went; what the person noticed when practicing mindfulness; any discoveries; and drawing out next steps. Facilitators seek to be consistently accepting of however much or little home practice people describe, and steadfastly encouraging of what people can do. The focus in this part of the session is on mindfulness practice, and facilitators need to shape the discussion when the conversation digresses.

Guiding Mindfulness Practices

The core mindfulness practice (discussed in Chapter 4) is completed twice per session. We provide a number of audio recordings to help you learn to guide mindfulness for people with psychosis. One recording (Track 1) closely follows the core mindfulness practice, and another (Track 6) is the brief practice used in the optional pre-program meeting. These recordings will give you a sense of the tone and pace that we have found works best in these groups, as well as the content of the guidance provided in the practices.

While the structure and script remain the same for the core mindfulness practice described above, there is some room for minor adjustments. With experience, you may bring in some of your own phrases and language when guiding the core mindfulness practice. You may also decide to make minor adaptations—for example, to emphasize the session theme, to respond to a live issue (such as hopelessness or frustration expressed by group members), or to shorten the second practice if time is tight. With this in mind, we have created four additional audio recordings for your use (Tracks 2–5). These additional recordings illustrate how you might make these minor adaptations to the core mindfulness practice. Track 2: "Core mindfulness practice—bringing in some of your own phrases and language," Track 3: "Core mindfulness practice—emphasizing the session theme," Track 4: "Core mindfulness practice—shortening the practice," and Track 5: "Core mindfulness practice—responding to a live issue" are intended to illustrate how you might make minor adaptations when guiding mindfulness in group sessions, to bring in your own phrasing, emphasize the session theme, shorten the practice if pressed for time, or respond to a live issue, respectively. These adjustments are optional and it is also fine, especially when learning the program, to stick with the written script.

If it is occasionally not possible to guide mindfulness practices yourself in sessions (e.g., if the lead facilitator is absent), it is fine to play an audio recording—your own or one of ours (specifically, Track 1 or Track 2). If it is not possible to make your own recording to share with group members to support their home practice, you may wish to download and share Track 1 or Track 2.

If there are two facilitators, each typically leads one practice and participates in the other, though it is fine for one person to guide all practices if preferred. It is also fine to have the script at hand when guiding mindfulness.

Having a second practice each session is important, even if slightly shorter than the first. A second practice shows that each practice is experienced differently, even if the words we use remain the same, and individuals who struggle with one practice get to see that they can be more settled during another. These differences are opportunities for reflection and acceptance of variation in mindfulness practice, which can in turn instill hope and motivation for practice during the week ahead.

Inquiry

Each mindfulness practice is followed by a guided *inquiry*, focused on validating people's experiences, guiding discovery, refining their understanding of mindfulness (and challenges faced during practice), and facilitating the group factors of universality, cohesion and belonging, hope, and being oneself more fully. Facilitators use reflections, summaries, and questions to retain focus and prevent drift.

In Chapter 5, we proposed a progression in how key metacognitive insights emerge over the course of the program. Session summaries reflect this progression, proposing unhelpful metacognitive beliefs to listen for, and helpful metacognitive insights to draw out during inquiry—metacognitive insights that have been discussed in one session can be rehearsed and reinforced in subsequent sessions. In practice, some participants will be further ahead than others, and we encourage facilitators to use this sequence flexibly.

When facilitating inquiry, we encourage people to decide how much they would like to share with the group. We make clear there is no requirement to share the details of difficult experiences or the *content* of difficult thoughts, voices, and images if this feels too uncomfortable or exposing. Our focus is on how these experiences affect us—how we feel and how we react, and how it feels if we can step back when they are happening and allow them to come and go without reacting. We usually remind people of this once or twice over the 8-week program.

Common Challenges to Mindfulness Practice

An important aspect of inquiry is drawing out and addressing challenges to practicing mindfulness during sessions (which are likely to occur during home practice, too). The guidance notes for each of the four pairs of sessions include a table of common challenges given the stage of the program, and suggestions for helpful facilitator responses. As a general guide, helpful responses usually recommend one or more of the following:

- Validate and normalize the challenge (e.g., "*Yes, it can be hard when our mind is busy and jumps around. Did anyone else notice this?*").
- Make specific or contextualize the challenge (e.g., "*So during the first practice . . .*").
- Address any misunderstandings about mindfulness practice.
- Look for moments of mindfulness—what did the person notice?
- Guide discovery (e.g., of metacognitive insights).
- Build universality, cohesion, and hope.
- Encourage and strengthen attitudinal qualities of kindness, self-compassion, and acceptance.

As with the emergence of metacognitive insights, there will be variability in when challenges to practice first present and many will come up repeatedly through the course of the program. We therefore once again encourage facilitators to use their judgment and be flexible when using these tables.

Inquiry following the second practice may be briefer and is an opportunity to reinforce any metacognitive insights articulated in the inquiry after the first practice. Toward the end of the inquiry after the second practice, facilitators may ask participants to name one thing they have learned that stands out for them. This can be done in pairs or as a group. Time permitting, facilitators may offer their own brief reflection on what has been shared.

Psychoeducation

Mindfulness groups involve very little didactic teaching, and never more than a few minutes at a time. In each session, we briefly introduce a topic linked to the session theme with relevant illustrative examples, ideally drawn from recent group discussion. To facilitate learning, we then invite group members to reflect on the topic, drawing on their direct experience. We check whether the material made sense, draw out any commonalities in people's reflections, and then briefly summarize key learning from psychoeducation.

Closing the Session and Home Practice

We encourage, though do not require, that group members do their own home practice. Each session closes with recommendations for members to try formal (core mindfulness practice) and informal practice (prompts for moments of mindfulness) prior to the next session. When possible, we recommend facilitators share an audio recording of themselves guiding the core mindfulness practice as group members find this supports home practice (following the script in Appendix 9.1). However, if you prefer, you may download and share the recording "Core mindfulness practice" (Track 1 at *www.guilford.com/chadwick-materials*). We end the session with warm and authentic gratitude for people's attendance and participation, and encouragement for the week ahead.

Supporting Behavior Change

As group members come to experience greater choice, acceptance, and empowerment in daily life, we find that most begin spontaneously reporting valued behavioral changes around Sessions 3 to 4. We support and encourage this at both the weekly check-in and in our closing remarks, linking this "reclaiming our lives" to increased mindfulness and self-acceptance in daily life. If by Session 4 an individual is not yet reporting small, though meaningful behavioral change, then we may more actively support them with this during periods of reflective discussion. The focus on valued behavior change increases in Sessions 7 and 8, with the theme "Taking mindful steps toward personal recovery."

Session Handouts

Each session includes a written handout. In preparing this guidance, we noticed a tension between the benefits of pre-prepared handouts and a wish for personalized summaries written after sessions. We have opted for pre-prepared handouts (available at *www.guilford.com/chadwick-materials*), because these are useful in reinforcing key learning and the process of change over the course of the program. We also recognize that most health care clinicians and mindfulness facilitators have limited time to generate materials. Each handout includes space for group members to add any points that were particularly important to them, which can be added at the close of the session (when facilitators may assist) or later at home. Handouts also have space for reflections following mindfulness practice over the week, to encourage practice and anticipate the next session.

9

Sessions 1 and 2: Stepping Back

At the start of the program, people commonly have concerns both about learning mindfulness and about being in a group. In relation to learning mindfulness, many people expect that they will not be able to *do mindfulness*, and will be judged for *getting it wrong.* In relation to being in a group, people may come with the metacognitive belief that "*I am fundamentally different, set apart, alone, even in this group.*" These fears create a lack of psychological safety.

In these opening sessions, facilitators work to engender hope and confidence in group members that "*Maybe I can learn mindfulness*" and "*Maybe I could fit in and belong here.*" Encouraging a sense that "*Maybe this is for me*" is underpinned by facilitators' embodiment of the core attitudinal qualities of authenticity, acceptance, and trust—in group members, mindfulness, and the process of change.

The theme for Sessions 1 and 2 is *stepping back*. People's confidence in practicing mindfulness comes from experiencing (1) moments of catching themselves lost in reactivity, then stepping back and letting go of reactions; (2) moments of decentered awareness of breathing and other sensations; and (3) emerging metacognitive insights about the impact of distressing habitual reactions and mindful responding. This learning usually starts with fleeting experiences of stepping back from reactivity to distressing psychosis during mindfulness practices.

Alongside this, a sense of safety and belonging develop from feeling that one's contributions are accepted and valued, as well as an emerging sense of universality with others in the group. People are beginning to experience and understand how mindfulness and being part of the group could be helpful as a new way of relating to psychosis.

Facilitating Group Factors in Sessions 1 and 2

For people with current psychosis, it takes considerable courage and effort to get to initial group sessions, stay until the end, and then travel home. In addition to anxiety about meeting new people, the feelings that trouble them day-to-day—such as fear, shame, guilt, frustration, and despair—will arise in the group. As a result, intrusive voices, images, paranoia, and other psychosis sensations are often strong. During the early sessions, group members' concentration waxes and wanes, given this emotional load.

The first two sessions focus on enabling people to get to know one another, and introducing mindfulness as a way to step back from psychosis and center awareness in the breath and body. Importantly, group members are forming an impression of the facilitators as people just as much as they are gauging other group members and mindfulness practice. We encourage facilitators to lean into the foundational therapist qualities of authenticity, acceptance, and trust (see Chapter 6), particularly when feeling uncertain.

In terms of cultivating group processes in Sessions 1 and 2, facilitators seek to foster the beginnings of all four key group factors: universality, cohesion and belonging, hope, and being myself more fully. While individuals differ in the degree to which these are experienced in these early sessions, some combination usually supports engagement with the program and a growing sense that the group may be safe and beneficial.

Universality

Universality is the recognition that we are all alike, and in the context of mindfulness for psychosis groups, that others have similar experiences. Universality is subjectively the most important group factor for people attending these groups (Chadwick et al., 2005, 2009). This initially comes from hearing that others also experience distressing psychosis, and have faced difficult life events and circumstances, leading to the possibility that "*Maybe I am not different.*" With careful facilitation, universality can emerge from the first sessions, in recognition of shared daily struggle to live and cope with psychosis and, for many, the impact of past trauma. As facilitators, we draw out and emphasize commonalities, while valuing people's differences. The beginnings of universality often emerge during inquiry, when facilitators actively look for and highlight common experiences of struggle in living with psychosis.

Cohesion

Cohesion describes a sense of belonging in the group. Meeting new people is a big step for most group members. People may hear omnipotent, malevolent voices, see disturbing images, and experience paranoia, grandiosity, or confusion during group discussions and mindfulness practices. Anxiety, fear, shame, and other difficult emotions may be present. This all makes connection with others, and therefore group cohesion, difficult.

Our intention in these initial sessions is to ensure that the group feels safe enough for people to start connecting with one another and try the mindfulness practices. The beginnings of group cohesion primarily come from the active listening, validation, and nonjudgmental acceptance of facilitators. We can show this in always finding something to value in what people share. We are also attentive to moments when group members show one another interest, kindness, and acceptance.

Hope

Hope arises from glimpses of universality and group cohesion. For many people new to mindfulness groups, feeling overwhelmed by psychosis and self-doubt dominate day-to-day life and restrict hope. Hope is about the possibility that "*Maybe I can do this*" and "*Maybe I'm not different*" and what might follow. As facilitators, we expect to hold and embody hope in people's ability to engage in mindfulness, and the therapeutic potential of this way of relating to psychosis. Given the nature of psychosis, many people's experiences of past interpersonal trauma, and the likelihood of previous iatrogenic harms, we are careful to express hope sensitively, and avoid cheerleading or setting high expectations for change that may undermine trust. Our experience is that group members recognize our quiet confidence in them, in mindfulness, and in the group, and that this is sufficient in these early sessions.

Being Myself More Fully

The fourth key group process that we actively seek to foster is for people to be themselves *more fully*. Many people avoid discussing experiences of psychosis, trauma, and exclusion, even with friends and family, due to shame and fear of being judged, rejected, or viewed as dangerous. Ending this silence is a vital first step in being more fully oneself. This usually involves talking more openly about the impact of living with distressing psychosis. As facilitators, we create opportunities for each person to share something of their experience, even if just that "*Life is hard*" or "*The voices are difficult.*" Having found the courage to share something about themselves, group members experience being validated and accepted by others in the group. Being oneself more fully in the group is a crucial step toward self-acceptance.

SESSION GUIDANCE

Sessions 1 and 2 Structure

1. Opening the session
2. *Session 1:* Group agreements

   Session 2: Review mindfulness practice over the week—formal practice and moments of mindfulness
3. First core mindfulness practice
4. Inquiry focused on first practice
5. *Session 1 psychoeducation:* (a) reacting to psychosis, (b) mindfulness might help, (c) learning together as a group

   Session 2 psychoeducation: (a) reacting to psychosis, (b) moving from reactivity to letting go—stepping back

[Optional break]

6. Second core mindfulness practice
7. Inquiry focused on second practice and session learning points
8. Closing the session and home practice

Handouts/Materials

- Session handout
- Audio recording of core mindfulness practice (either your own recording of the "Core mindfulness practice," or the version we provide online in Track 1; see Appendix 9.1).

Opening the Session

We start the first session by welcoming everyone and recognizing that simply being here is hard for some:

> "*OK, let's make a start. Welcome everyone. It's good to see you all here today. My name is . . . and I'm one of the facilitators of the group. We know that traveling to a new group and meeting new people can be stressful, so well done for getting here. To get started, it would be great if each of you would say just your first name, and how you found the journey here today.*"

Even at this opening stage, we can emphasize universality in feelings of anxiety or ambivalence about coming to the group, emphasizing how this is understandable and normal. We then introduce the 8-week program:

> "*So, again, welcome. This is an 8-week mindfulness group for people struggling to cope with difficult voices, images, thoughts, and worries* [adapt given knowledge of the group]. *Mindfulness groups like this have been running for over 20 years. Mindfulness can help us learn to cope better with difficult experiences and have some more choice and control in our lives. You don't need to have practiced mindfulness before—we will learn together. Learning with people who have similar experiences can help you become more accepting of yourself and feel less alone.*"

We then cover practical details: duration of sessions, whether there will be breaks, location of toilets, which exits to use in case of emergency, and so on. We give explicit permission for people to leave the room if needed:

> "*Just to say, it's fine if you need to leave the room at any time. Please leave as quietly as you can, especially if we are practicing mindfulness,* [and if there are two group facilitators] *and one of us will come out just to check that you're OK.*"

In Session 2, we welcome participants back to the group, with brief introductions for any newcomers and a reminder of the group agreements (see below). We then outline the structure of the session:

"Welcome, it's good to see you all. This is the second of our eight sessions. As before, we'll do two mindfulness practices today and have some discussion about how they went and how mindfulness might be useful to you."

Group Agreements

Setting group agreements is an important step in creating psychological safety and enabling people to begin to express and be themselves in the group. This is done in the first session and rehearsed briefly in the second. A list of group agreements is set collaboratively. We recommend facilitators ensure these agreements include commitments to:

- Treating everyone in the group with kindness and respect
- Learning about and practicing mindfulness
- Confidentiality—not talking about group members outside the group

Check-In on Mindfulness Practice (Second Session)

From Session 2 onward, opening the session flows into reflective discussion of mindfulness practice over the past week. It can help to acknowledge the likelihood of past trauma, while clarifying that the focus in the group is on current experience—for example:

"We know that many people experience difficult voices, paranoia, images, and other sensations because of past trauma. While in this group we will focus on how things are currently and how mindfulness can support your well-being and recovery; we want to acknowledge the impact of trauma for many of you."

It can take a few sessions of gentle shaping for people to focus on mindfulness-related feedback. For example, when group members describe having had a difficult week, the facilitator might say:

"So, it's been a tough week, lots going on for you, Sam. Were there any moments when mindfulness or the group came to mind?"

We ask whether people have listened to the audio recordings of the core mindfulness practice, and about any moments of mindfulness in daily life (see Chapter 4):

"To start off we want to check in on mindfulness practices over the past week. Did anyone manage the 10-minute mindfulness practice this week?"

People usually describe a mix of formal practice (using the recordings) and informal practice (noticing moments of reaction or mindfulness in their daily lives). Our aim is to respond warmly to each person, expressing interest in what it was like to practice, formally and informally, and encouraging those who haven't yet practiced:

"That's fine, it can take time to embed mindfulness in our daily lives—it's great to see you here today."

During the check-in, we validate stressful experiences (1) emphasizing universality (e.g., "*Sandra, Marik, it sounds like you both had a hard time with voices this week*"), (2) clarifying any ongoing misunderstandings about mindfulness (e.g., "*So you found that when practicing mindfulness, sometimes your mind settled and sometimes the difficult thoughts kept coming up. Thanks Marik, that's an important point—sometimes our minds become a little quieter with mindfulness and sometimes the mind remains very busy*"), and (3) addressing barriers to home practice while accepting that some will do little or none.

Depending on the feedback, we can link discussion to the session theme, stepping back:

"Many of you noticed this week how often you get caught up struggling with difficult voices, images, and thoughts, and how distressing this can be. Last week, we talked about how it's normal and understandable to get lost in struggling with these sensations and today we'll talk more about how coming to this group and practicing stepping back may be helpful to you."

Finally, from Session 2, we draw people's attention to the possibility of being mindful of enjoyable as well as stressful experiences:

"We have talked quite a bit about bringing mindfulness to unpleasant and frightening experiences, such as voices or difficult thoughts and images,

but we can be mindful of anything we experience—pleasant as well as unpleasant. Did anyone have any moments over the last week where they were really present and mindful of a moment of joy or of connection, maybe with another person, a pet, or in nature?"

Usually someone responds, but if not, we would offer a simple example from our own week to model this application of mindfulness in daily life, and emphasize how important it is to attend to these moments, as well as unpleasant ones:

"I had quite a stressful week, but I saw my young nephew a few days ago. We went for a short walk—he's just five, likes to hold my hand, and is interested in everything around him. It was lovely just walking along with him for those few minutes, and I noticed my body relaxing."

Introducing and Guiding the Core Mindfulness Practices

The core mindfulness practice was developed specifically for people with distressing psychosis. This exercise is practiced twice each session, following the script in Appendix 9.1. It begins with focused awareness on bodily sensations and breathing, and then encourages opening attention to *choiceless awareness* of present experience, including psychosis and other sensations. When decentered awareness is lost, the guidance encourages people gently to reconnect with their breathing and then open out again. The guidance intentionally directs people's attention to how it feels to be caught in habitual reactions, to step back and let go of reacting, and to rest attention in a decentered awareness of breathing and other sensations. Before starting, we encourage readers to revisit Chapter 4, which describes the practice in detail.

At Session 1, we typically introduce the first practice in this way:

"It's difficult to really understand what mindfulness is without doing it. So, let's practice together for a few minutes. [Modeling posture] *If we can, it helps to sit upright and rest our feet on the floor. If you feel comfortable in doing so, gently allow your eyes to close; this just cuts down on the distractions around us. If you need to keep your eyes open, that's fine, just rest your gaze on the floor in front of you. Likewise, if you need to open your eyes during the practice, just allow your gaze to rest on the floor in*

front of you. If you need to get up and leave the room, that's fine; please just be as quiet as possible. I will guide us through the practice. Please be silent during the practice, and afterward we can talk about how it went."

When guiding the second practice each session, facilitators may weave in one or two additional phrases or emphasize existing phrases that capture important points from inquiry following the first practice. For example, at this early stage in the group program, people can feel frustration at how little time they are mindful, perhaps seldom noticing their breathing or even the guidance. It is also important to emphasize and repeat sections of guidance that encourage kindness and self-acceptance, using phrases that (1) emphasize that we are all doing the best we can (e.g., "*as best we can,*" "*if we can*"); (2) normalize getting lost in reaction and encouraging nonjudgment when this happens (e.g., "*If you find you've been lost, there's no need to judge yourself, we all get lost in this way*"); (3) convey the importance of gentle concentration (e.g., "*It's important not to try too hard to be mindful. If we try too hard, we just make ourselves tense and stressed—see if you can find a level of gentle concentration*"); and (4) highlight that it is always possible, in this moment, to come back to the breath and begin again (e.g., "*When you notice you've been lost in reaction—that's fine, that's just what our minds do—gently bringing your attention back to the breath to begin again*").

Occasionally someone speaks aloud during a practice, perhaps commenting on or reacting to what they are noticing. If this happens more than once, we weave a brief comment into the guidance, such as:

"Trying as best we can to be silent for the practice. It can be helpful to note to ourselves—silently in our own mind—what we are aware of, so maybe noting 'voices,' or 'thoughts' as they arise."

Facilitating the Two Periods of Inquiry

Mindfulness practice brings people into direct, conscious contact with present-moment experience. Guidance during practice encourages a decentered awareness of experiences that arise, and the specific qualities of these experiences. Inquiry following practice draws out key learning from these moments.

Each guided practice is followed by some minutes of inquiry (see Chapter 5). The first period of inquiry follows and focuses on the first mindfulness practice. The second inquiry follows the second mindfulness practice, and pulls together key learning from the entire session.

Inquiry involves validation, supporting universality and other group factors, and guiding discovery of metacognitive insights—about psychosis experience, sources of distress (habitual reactivity) and well-being (mindful responding), and the self. At this stage, people start to notice periods lost in distressing reaction, and rarer moments of decentered awareness; inquiry focuses on learning from both. Facilitators embody authenticity, acceptance, and trust, and always find value in what people say. Not everyone needs to speak during each inquiry and we avoid a turn-taking approach; people can benefit from just listening.

Inquiry in early sessions is also a time to address common misconceptions about mindfulness—for example, that the aim is to stop unpleasant voices, images, or thoughts, or create an empty mind, or achieve a state of physical relaxation. These misunderstandings often need to be addressed a few times.

Session 1: We open the first period of inquiry saying something like "*The first thing to say is 'Well done.' It's not easy to practice mindfulness for the first time. It can feel worrying or scary, but you did it. How was that for you?*" If reflections remain quite general (e.g., "*It was fine*"), then more specific prompts can be helpful, such as "*What did anyone notice?*" or "*Did anyone have any difficult voices, images, thoughts, or other unusual experiences during the practice? How was that?*" to draw attention to direct experience and support discovery.

Session 2: From Session 2 onward, each period of inquiry begins with an open question to the group, such as "*How was that practice?*" Facilitators draw attention to moments of direct experience during practice and use these as opportunities for validating, building universality and other group factors, and guiding discovery. Facilitators balance being open and responsive to whatever group members raise, with shaping the discussion in line with (1) the session theme, (2) the two-circles model (see Chapter 2, Figure 2.1), and (3) the core process of change (see Chapter 3).

In each session, we close the second period of inquiry by inviting group members to share one thing that they have learned or that stands out for them from the session. We might also offer a brief final reflection or summary of our own:

> "*Today you have all done your first two practices; well done. You are getting a sense of what mindfulness is and we've begun to see some of the things we have in common.*"

Focusing on Moments of Mindfulness Practice That Support Learning

In these early sessions we are not expecting people to stop reacting to psychosis sensations. Much of people's time will be spent lost in habitual reactivity (the left side of the two-circles model), and our aim is to facilitate awareness and learning from this as well as from any moments of decentered awareness (the right side of the model), drawing out how these two ways of relating feel in the body and mind, and emotionally.

As described in Chapter 5, the focus during inquiry and other reflective discussion evolves session by session in line with the two-circles model and the core process of change in mindfulness for psychosis. In these sessions, we listen for and ask questions to reinforce a gentle, compassionate approach to mindfulness practice, awareness of the impact of habitual reactions, and attention to any moments of mindful responding.

Attitude Toward Practice

We encourage, and may model through careful self-disclosure, a compassionate approach to mindfulness practice and ourselves. We encourage people to concentrate gently and not try too hard. We normalize difficulty maintaining decentered awareness, which also builds universality and invites self-compassion (e.g., "*Yes, we all find it hard to stay in the present moment*"). To foster hope and motivation, we emphasize that no matter how many times we lose present-moment awareness, it is always possible to step back, refocus on our breathing, and begin again (and again).

Guiding Discovery about Habitual Reactions

During inquiry, we take time to draw out how it feels to be caught in reactivity (the left side of the two-circles model), with no expectation of change. As facilitators, we emphasize the value of recognizing when we are caught in habitual, distressing reaction—getting to know how this feels in the body and mind, and emotionally. From the first session, facilitators focus on *learning to recognize habitual reactions*, again with no expectation that people suddenly stop reacting. Facilitators draw out and emphasize the universality of these instinctive reactions to unpleasant and frightening sensations. For example:

> "*So, Mo, you're noticing that when these frightening thoughts come up—that your neighbors are watching you, planning to hurt you—you*

understandably get into a struggle in your mind, trying to work out if this is true, but this leaves you feeling even more tense, more frightened. Has anyone else had the experience of reacting to their voices, images, or thoughts in ways that leave them feeling worse?"

We build universality and take any opportunities to guide discovery about the helpful metacognitive insights that "*We can all get locked into our mind—reacting to unpleasant and frightening experiences*" and "*Getting lost in reacting is distressing and exhausting.*"

Drawing Attention to Unhelpful Metacognitive Beliefs

From Session 2 onward, facilitators listen for and gently inquire about unhelpful metacognitive beliefs that maintain habitual ways of reacting, and any related self-judgments. These are usually implicit and can be drawn out with careful guided discovery. For example:

> *"You've said how hard it is to step back and let go of resisting. I wonder, do you have any fears about what might happen if you stop resisting or struggling against unpleasant voices?"*

If individuals are unsure of how to respond, it can be helpful to invite others to comment (e.g., "*That's OK, it can be hard to put these things into words. What do others think?*"). This can elicit one or more unhelpful metacognitive beliefs that underpin and maintain distressing reactivity to psychosis.

While these beliefs are not directly questioned or challenged by facilitators, drawing them out in the group can begin to lessen their hold, and prompt people to notice that their fears are not borne out during mindfulness practice. Facilitators comment on how many of us hold beliefs that keep us locked in avoidance, struggle, and judgment, even though these reactions aren't working well, thereby strengthening universality.

Moments of Mindful Responding

In these early sessions, in addition to learning from observing patterns of reactivity (the left side of the two-circles model), it is important that people experience some moments of mindful responding (the right side of the model). As facilitators, we listen for and highlight moments of decentered awareness of breathing, bodily sensations, or psychosis sensations. We draw out how the person felt in these moments. When people describe noticing psychosis sensations, we emphasize that any moments of noticing voices, images, thoughts, and other unpleasant sensations without reacting *are moments of mindfulness*. This helps people recognize that they are starting to engage with the practice (and addresses the misunderstanding that people are only being mindful when focused on their breathing).

Just two or three moments of decentered awareness during a 10-minute practice are sufficient to begin to instill hope and confidence in mindfulness practice. Guided discovery of new learning strengthens this emerging confidence and fosters motivation for practice. For example, with bodily awareness, many people are struck by how seldom they notice their body in daily life—"*I didn't realize how tense I was; I don't normally notice what's going on in my body, I'm just in my head.*"

Meeting Psychosis Sensations with Decentered Awareness—Illustrative Dialogue

A common misunderstanding is to assume that being mindful means focusing solely on the breath. We can help people recognize that meeting psychosis sensations with decentered awareness is just as much *being mindful* as decentered awareness of breathing. The core mindfulness practice encourages a *choiceless awareness* precisely so people learn that their attention does not need to remain fixed on their breathing. This common misunderstanding leaves people striving to pull their attention away from voices, images, thoughts, feelings, and other sensations, causing further distress and tension. The following dialogue illustrates how a facilitator might guide discovery about meeting psychosis sensations with decentered awareness:

MARIUS: I couldn't do it. The images were right here in my mind. I couldn't come back to the breathing—they were too strong. They won like they always do.

FACILITATOR: So you noticed the images were right here, center stage. Yes, that's exactly what mindfulness is, to be aware of our present experience. And then you tried to pull back to your breathing. Is that right?

MARIUS: Yeah. I tried to but they just got stronger and stronger. I couldn't do it.

FACILITATOR: OK. That's also important to notice—when you tried to pull your attention away, the images got stronger, and it got harder and harder to bring your awareness back to your breath. Is that right?

MARIUS: Yes, that's right, that's how it is.

FACILITATOR: This is a really important thing to notice or discover. It's almost like strong images and thoughts are pulling your attention toward them, and you are trying hard to pull your attention back to your breathing. Almost like in a tug-of-war.

CASS: You just can't ignore them, however hard you try, not when they're so strong.

FACILITATOR: Right, so what you are finding is that when images, thoughts, and voices are strong and in the center of your awareness, you can't pull your attention away. And if you try to pull your attention away at these times, it's stressful and they just get stronger. So, what can we do? What would be a mindful way to respond when voices, thoughts, and images are strong, and right there in the center of our awareness?

MARIUS: Just let them. Let them be there.

FACILITATOR: Let them! Yes. Mindfulness is about being aware of what is happening. So, if there are strong voices, thoughts, images, whatever it is, we can allow them to be in the center of our awareness for a while. Allow them to be there without reacting, without struggling.

CASS: Let them be there, not fight with them—try to anyway?

FACILITATOR: Yes. As best you can, observe them without reacting and without trying to pull your attention away. And when they fade into the background, or pass entirely, that's the time to gently bring our awareness back to the breathing.

Common Challenges to Practice at Sessions 1 and 2

Common challenges in these early sessions center on self-doubt ("*I can't do it*") and doubt about the value of mindfulness ("*It won't work*," "*It can't work*"). Common challenges often arise at this stage in the program, typically during inquiry, alongside linked metacognitive beliefs. Importantly, no particular response is *right*; facilitators will respond flexibly in line with the two-circles model and the core process of change. See the following table for common challenges and possible responses that often arise at this stage.

Common Challenges Arising in Sessions 1 and 2, and Possible Responses

Challenges	Examples	Unhelpful metacognitive beliefs and judgments	Possible responses from facilitators
Concerns about not being able to do *mindfulness*	*"I had too much going on in my head, I couldn't do it."*	*"I should be able to do this, I should be able to control my mind."*	Validate, normalize, and emphasize universality. *"Everybody's mind is busy and jumps around. I know mine does! Did others notice that?"*
	"I can't do this, it's too difficult."	*"There's something wrong with me, something lacking—I haven't got what it takes to be mindful."*	Look for moments of mindfulness; what *did* the person notice? *"Were there any moments, even just for a second or two, when you were able to notice your breathing, or the thoughts or voices?"* *"Great, so there were moments when you noticed your breathing, and when you noticed the voices were there. That's a great start!"*
	"The voices and images were too strong, they always win."	*"The voices and images are too powerful, I'll never be able to change how I react."*	Instill hope in a way that is likely to be heard. *"Yes, it takes time to learn mindfulness. You've been coping and reacting in these ways for a long time, and it will take a while to learn to step back."*
	"I couldn't concentrate, I'm not up to it."	*"I'll never be able to do it, I'll never get it right. I never get anything right."*	Validate and make it specific or contextualize. *"So, it was really hard to concentrate today. That's understandable. The voices were strong and you've been anxious about the group and slept badly last night. It usually gets easier, once you're more used to being in the group."*

Concerns about mindfulness not *working*	*"It didn't work, the images are still here, I can't get rid of them."*	*"Mindfulness can't help—the only thing that can help is getting rid of them."*	Validate and guide discovery. *"It sounds as if that was tough—well-done for sticking with it. You said there were some moments when you were able to let the images be there without having to block them out. How does it feel to be able to do that some of the time, to be able to watch them come and go without reacting?"*
		"Watching my breath can't get rid of them."	Normalize and emphasize universality. *"There are times for us all when it feels too much. Choosing to open your eyes for a while during that practice sounds like the right thing to have done. Were you able to reconnect with the practice at all?"*
	"It was too much, I had to open my eyes, the thoughts were too much."	*"If I let them in, I won't be able to cope."*	Look for moments of mindfulness and guide discovery. *"Were there any moments when the voices were not there, or faded a little into the background?"* *"So, you noticed one time how they faded and then stopped. Stepping back and noticing them fade is mindfulness. We can build on that. When they faded and stopped, where did your attention move to?"*
			Instill hope in a way that can be heard and address misunderstandings. *"You're right, mindfulness doesn't get rid of difficult voices and images. It doesn't stop us from having difficult thoughts and feelings; we all have them. It's about learning to step back and cope in a different way—not always getting lost in reaction and struggle, instead learning to have a little more choice, and not feeling so overwhelmed and exhausted all the time."* *"Focusing on our breathing helps us step back when things are stressful and difficult. It can become like an anchor, grounding us in our breath and body."*

Psychoeducation in Sessions 1 and 2

After the first practice and inquiry, the psychoeducation component of the session focuses on a key aspect of mindfulness for psychosis in line with the session theme. Psychoeducation involves *very little didactic talking*, typically 2–3 minutes at most. Facilitators briefly introduce the topic, illustrate this by drawing on earlier discussion (e.g., during inquiry), and then invite group discussion, during which we listen for shared experiences and check understanding. Session 1 psychoeducation focuses on three linked points: (1) reacting to psychosis, (2) mindfulness might help, and (3) learning together in a group.

Reacting to Psychosis

Here, we highlight that habitual reactions to psychosis are common, understandable, and distressing (anticipating the left side of the two-circles model). For example:

> "*You've begun talking about how hard it is to live with distressing voices, images, thoughts, and other sensations, and just how overwhelmed many of you are feeling. You spend lots of time pushing these experiences away or getting caught up in struggling, fighting, and judging yourselves. These ways of coping are common and understandable but don't work well for you and are exhausting.*"

Mindfulness Might Help

The second point highlights that mindfulness may present an alternative and more helpful way of coping (anticipating the right side of the two-circles model). For example:

> "*Today we've begun to practice mindfulness. Mindfulness won't stop difficult voices, images, thoughts, or other sensations from happening. Mindfulness is about learning to cope with these experiences in a different way. We can learn to pause, step back, focus on our breath and body, and not always have to get lost in struggle and reaction when things are stressful. Mindfulness can give us more choice.*"

Learning Together in a Group

The third point to highlight in the first session is that the group can learn mindfulness together:

> *"Being in a group with people who have similar experiences can really help. When you're feeling overwhelmed with psychosis, it's easy to feel different and alone. Here, in a group with people who have similar problems, you can see that you are not different, you are not alone, that we all have things in common, and can support one another. [Pause] Does this make sense? Does anyone have any comments or questions about what I've said, or about mindfulness?"*

Session 2 psychoeducation builds on these and focuses on (1) reacting to psychosis, and (2) moving from reactivity to letting go—stepping back.

Reacting to Psychosis

We highlight again that people are spending a lot of time reacting to psychosis (with avoidance, rumination, worry, confrontation, and judgment), and that this is normal and understandable—we all react in these ways to unpleasant and unwanted experiences. Additionally, reacting in these ways is distressing and exhausting.

Moving from Reactivity to Letting Go—Stepping Back

Following this, if we can catch ourselves reacting to unpleasant sensations, it is sometimes possible to step back and let go of reacting and bring awareness back to the breath. Letting go of reacting often feels calming:

> *"We've talked about how you are all spending a lot of time reacting to difficult voices, images, thoughts, and feelings—maybe trying to avoid them, or resisting and fighting them, or worrying about them. Today, we want to spend a few minutes pulling together what we are learning about these ways of reacting to difficult sensations. First, we've found that it's completely normal to react in these ways. We all do it—when an unpleasant thought or image comes into my mind, my immediate reaction is to try to avoid it, distract myself somehow. We all try to avoid or resist threatening*

experiences. Second, we've seen that these ways of reacting aren't really working for you—Marius, you said they don't stop the images; Cass, you said that shouting back or resisting the voices makes them worse. These automatic ways of reacting—avoiding, worrying, fighting—leave you exhausted. Finally, we've started to see that there is an alternative way of relating to difficult voices, images, thoughts, and other sensations. Many of you have had moments of stepping back, letting go of reacting, and focusing on your breathing. How does it feel when you let go of struggling and come back to focusing on your breathing?"

Closing the Session, Home Practice, and Handouts

Commitment to home practice is not a requirement in mindfulness for psychosis groups. We invite people to try the core mindfulness practice at home over the coming week (either your own recording of the "Core mindfulness practice" (Track 1), or the version we provide on the accompanying web page at *www.guilford.com/chadwick-materials*). We note that mindfulness is a skill and, like any skill, takes time and practice. We acknowledge that home practice is sometimes not possible and ask people to do what they can each week, and even if they aren't able to practice, to please come back for the next session. The session handouts cover key learning, encourage formal and informal practice, and have space for people to note any comments or reflections from the session and week ahead (see Handouts 1 and 2, below).

We spend a couple of minutes distributing and describing the session handout. This includes highlighting formal and informal practice (*moments of mindfulness*). In the Session 1 handout, we suggest people practice this through *checking in on ourselves*:

"In addition to the 10-minute recording, try to notice any moments of mindfulness during the day. Moments of mindfulness are when we just pause and 'check in with ourselves'—tuning into sensations in the body and the flow of sensations as we breathe in and breathe out, just for a few moments. This can be done anywhere—maybe waiting for a bus, standing in a line, sitting at home. Consider putting a reminder on your phone or a card in your purse or wallet to prompt you to take a moment for mindfulness a few times a day."

In the Session 2 handout, we suggest people practice moments of mindfulness through noticing moments of joy and connection with other people:

> *"We've talked about how struggling with psychosis can dominate your life. This brings suffering and can make it hard to connect with other people and enjoy living. This week, as best you can, continue noticing moments of mindfulness in your daily life. You can continue with 'checking in with ourselves'—tuning into the sensations of breathing for a few moments, any time and any place. Additionally, try to open to moments of joy and connection—for example, with other people or nature when these arise."*

Just as we start each session by *meeting the person, not the problem,* we close sessions with warmth and authenticity—for example: *"It's been good to meet you all today and to have started this group together. We hope you each have a good week and look forward to seeing you all next time."*

APPENDIX 9.1. Core Mindfulness Practice

Opening Phase

1. Let's start by taking a moment to sit comfortably in the chair, sitting in an upright, relaxed position with your feet resting on the floor. If it feels comfortable, allow your eyes to close, or if you prefer, rest your gaze on the floor in front of you. It is easy to get locked in our mind, lost in thinking, so we begin mindfulness by bringing awareness to our body. It can help to bring our awareness to a point of contact, so if you can, gently bring your awareness to the soles of your feet on the floor. Really connect with the sensations in this place in your body—maybe notice feelings of temperature or pressure. Maybe warmth or cold.

2. Sometimes, if we really connect with the sensations in the soles of our feet, we can notice tingling sensations that move around, come and go. We can see how nothing stays in awareness for long.

3. Now gently bring your awareness up into your legs. Just notice whatever sensations are present right now in this part of your body, maybe notice the pressure of the chair, or the feeling of clothing against your skin. Don't worry if you can't notice any sensations in a part of your body; this is quite normal. Now, move your awareness to your upper body: your torso, arms, and hands. Just notice whatever sensations are happening right now in this moment. And across your shoulders. We often carry a lot of tension in our shoulders; if you become aware that your shoulders are tense, see if it is possible to relax them a little. Bring your awareness to your face, scalp, and inside your mouth.

4. Now bring your awareness gently to the sensations in your body as you breathe in and as you breathe out. Find that place in your body where you can notice the sensations as you breathe in and breathe out, where it's comfortable for you to rest your awareness. This might be noticing the rise and fall of your tummy or chest as you breathe in and out, or you may prefer to focus on the tips of your nostrils, noticing the sensations as the cooler air comes in and the slightly warmer air goes out.

5. We are not trying to change or control our breathing in any way. Mindfulness is about experiencing things just as they are. So, as best we can, experience one in-breath from its beginning to end just as it is, and one out-breath from its beginning to end just as it is.

(continued)

From *Mindfulness for Psychosis: A Group Therapy Approach*, by Paul Chadwick, Katherine Newman-Taylor, and Nicola Abba. Copyright © 2027 The Guilford Press. Permission to photocopy this material, or to download and print enlarged versions (*www.guilford.com/chadwick-materials*), is granted to purchasers of this book for personal use or use with clients; see copyright page for details.

Core Mindfulness Practice *(page 2 of 2)*

Middle Phase

6. We are not trying to force our attention to stay on the breathing. What we all find is that our awareness moves naturally to other things: sounds, thoughts, voices, images, worries, judgments, feelings. For these few minutes, if we can, allow each of these sensations to come fully into awareness, and then allow them to pass or fade into the background, without reacting to them. Each time we allow our awareness gently to return and rest again in the sensations of breathing.

7. You may find that difficult voices, images, thoughts, feelings, and other sensations come back again a few moments later. This is what happens. As best we can, each time we patiently allow difficult voices, images, thoughts, and feelings to come fully into awareness and then to pass or fade, without getting lost or caught up in them, without thinking about them or trying to work them out. In the spaces between the voices, images, thoughts, and other sensations, allow awareness to gently return to rest in the sensations of breathing.

8. Often, we find we have been lost, maybe struggling with voices, caught up in rumination or worry. We all get lost like this. There is no need to judge yourself. When this happens, as best we can, we notice how it feels in the body, how it feels emotionally, to let go of this struggle and reconnect with the sensations of breathing. Just rest awareness in the sensations as we breathe in and as we breathe out.

9. Remember that we are not trying to get rid of voices, images, thoughts, and feelings. We are not trying to create an empty mind. We are practicing being with difficult voices, images, thoughts, and sensations in a different way: allowing them to come fully into awareness and pass or fade without having to react, without having to struggle or fight or analyze.

10. If even once you are able to allow a difficult voice, thought, or image to come fully into awareness and pass or fade without reacting—if you can do this even once—notice how that feels in your body and mind, and emotionally in your mind.

Closing Phase

11. For the last minute, as best we can, be open to whatever sensations arise, whether pleasant or unpleasant or neutral. Allow all experiences to come fully into awareness and then pass or fade without reacting.

12. When you are ready, gently open your eyes and settle back into the room.

Mindfulness Group: Session 1 Handout

Well-done on joining the group and starting to learn mindfulness! Here's how people from previous groups have found it helped them:

Meeting Others with Similar Experiences

"It's good talking to other people who have the same sort of problems as you. Just to know you're not on your own, other people are going through similar things."—ANNA

Learning How to *Step Back*

"Mindfulness helps—learning to manage the paranoia and voices by taking a step back. I have more control now. I've learned I have a choice—to take a step back." —DOM

Having More Choice and Control in Life

"The big change is seeing I have a choice. I don't have to go down the same path every time. I can choose to go a different way. I can actually go out and start living again."—MAY

Feeling Better about Myself

"You learn to feel better about yourself, more accepting of yourself. I'm starting to like myself again."—SAM

It can help to write down one or two things you learned in Session 1:

____

____

____

____

____

(continued)

From *Mindfulness for Psychosis: A Group Therapy Approach*, by Paul Chadwick, Katherine Newman-Taylor, and Nicola Abba. Copyright © 2027 The Guilford Press. Permission to photocopy this material, or to download and print enlarged versions (*www.guilford.com/chadwick-materials*), is granted to purchasers of this book for personal use or use with clients; see copyright page for details.

Home Practice

Practicing mindfulness at home will help you learn mindfulness and use it in your daily life. We suggest you listen to the 10-minute guided mindfulness practice—each day if you can. See if you can find a time of day that works for you to sit quietly and listen to this.

We also recommend you try to notice any *moments of mindfulness* during the day. Moments of mindfulness are when we just pause and *check in with ourselves*—tuning into sensations in the body and the flow of sensations as we breathe in and breathe out, just for a few moments. This can be done anywhere—maybe waiting for a bus, standing in a line, sitting at home. Consider putting a reminder on your phone or a card in your purse or wallet to prompt you to take a moment for mindfulness a few times a day.

Both types of practice help us learn mindfulness and have more choice in how we live our lives.

Week 1 Diary

Some people find it helpful to jot down anything they notice or learn from practicing mindfulness between sessions. Feel free to make any notes here. If you'd like, you can share any of these reflections with the group in the next session.

Mindfulness Group: Session 2 Handout

We all react quickly and without thinking to unpleasant experiences like frightening thoughts, critical voices, and disturbing images—this is only natural as we are built to react to signs of threat.

Our instinctive reactions can include:

- Trying to avoid or block out unwanted thoughts, feelings, voices, and images
- Ruminating and worrying—going around and around in our head, trying to work it all out
- Confronting or fighting back
- Judging these experiences as bad or dangerous, and judging ourselves for having them

These instinctive reactions are often distressing and exhausting. Reacting doesn't work well when living with psychosis, and can make the voices, images, thoughts, and other sensations even stronger. This habit of getting stuck or lost in reacting also leaves little time and energy for what's important to us: the things and relationships we most value.

With mindfulness we can learn to respond differently to unpleasant sensations. We start learning mindfulness by:

- Noticing our usual reactions when they're happening
- Noticing the impact of these reactions on the body, mind, and emotions
- Learning to let go of these reactions and focus on the breath or body for a few moments

Letting go of reacting can be a relief and give strength—we'll talk more about this in the next session.

There will be many times this week when you react to difficult voices, images, thoughts, and other sensations. This is normal and understandable. As best you can, try not to judge yourselves for this. We know you are doing your best and it takes us all time to learn to respond differently to unpleasant experiences.

(continued)

From *Mindfulness for Psychosis: A Group Therapy Approach*, by Paul Chadwick, Katherine Newman-Taylor, and Nicola Abba. Copyright © 2027 The Guilford Press. Permission to photocopy this material, or to download and print enlarged versions (*www.guilford.com/chadwick-materials*), is granted to purchasers of this book for personal use or use with clients; see copyright page for details.

Home Practice

This week, as best you can:

- *Notice reactivity*—notice when you are reacting to unpleasant sensations and how this feels in your body and mind, and emotionally
- *Notice letting go*—notice any moments when you're able to let go of these reactions and focus on the breath for a few moments
- *Practice guided mindfulness*—listen to the 10-minute audio recording; have you found a time of day when this works for you?
- *Notice moments of mindfulness*—as well as *checking in with ourselves* (tuning into the sensations of breathing), try to experience moments of joy and connection fully when these arise

Please make a note of one or two things you learned in Session 2:

____

____

____

____

____

Week 2 Diary

Over the week, jot down anything you notice or learn from practicing mindfulness between sessions. You may wish to share your reflections with the group in the next session:

____

____

____

____

____

____

____

10

Sessions 3 and 4: Choosing How to Respond

The theme for Sessions 3 and 4 is *choice*, and specifically *choosing how to respond*. The choice is not between having or not having psychosis sensations, which most people have been striving for, unsuccessfully, for many years. The choice is between reacting habitually or stepping back and allowing these sensations to come into awareness and then pass or fade without reacting. In the first two sessions, most people have started to recognize their habitual reactions (avoiding, ruminating, worrying, confronting, judging), and how it feels to be caught in cycles of reactivity. Some have also experienced moments of decentered awareness of breathing, and of stepping back and letting go of reacting.

In Sessions 3 and 4, facilitators continue to draw out and contrast moments of distressing reactivity and mindful responding (the two-circles model; Chapter 2, Figure 2.1). Choosing to let go of habitual reactions and respond mindfully is rooted in the metacognitive understanding that "*Reacting creates suffering*," and that "*Responding mindfully reduces distress and feels calming, empowering.*" Starting to respond mindfully brings the possibility of a different way of living with psychosis, one in which people have a growing sense of choice, control, and power.

In addition to an emerging awareness of choice over how to relate to psychosis sensations, group members start to recognize that their habitual patterns of reactivity also apply to a range of other stressors, such as difficult interactions and day-to-day frustrations. We support people in recognizing and encouraging this broader application of the two-circles model of habitual reacting and mindful responding.

Facilitating Group Factors in Sessions 3 and 4

Universality

Participants are starting to feel more confident in a sense of shared experience with others, both in terms of their psychosis and their reactions to these sensations and other stressors. In Sessions 3 and 4 facilitators continue to draw out commonalities in both, and through guided discovery extend this to draw out universality in how it feels in the body and mind, and emotionally to (1) catch oneself reacting, step back, and choose to let go of reaction; (2) observe the breath, body sensations, and psychosis sensations; and (3) open to moments of joy and connection in daily life. Universality lies less in exact details of events, and more in the feelings, physical sensations, and learning that accompany these experiences, creating a sense of common humanity. This deepening sense of universality strengthens cohesion and hope and encourages people to express themselves more fully in the group.

Cohesion

For many, initial fears about safety and being judged or viewed as different are dissipating. A sense of safety, trust, and connection in the group emerge through growing universality, familiarity with the session structure, facilitators and other group members, and facilitators' embodiment of authenticity, acceptance, and trust. This builds motivation and commitment to persevere in the face of challenges, including doubts about mindfulness.

Facilitators listen for signs of group cohesion, often expressed as "*we . . .* " or "*the group*" and reflect this back using language that assumes a valued group identity (e.g., "*I'm struck by how many of you already look forward to our group meetings*" or "*I'm struck by your commitment to the group, coming today even after a difficult night with little sleep*"). As cohesion grows, people are more likely to address supportive and encouraging comments directly to each other. Facilitators listen for and validate expressions of kindness among group members.

Hope

With mindfulness practice comes experiential knowledge of the contrast between getting stuck in distressing reactivity and choosing to respond mindfully. This choice is empowering and instills hope, as people begin to see "*My role in alleviating distress and suffering*" (see Chapter 3). Hope in the therapeutic potential of mindfulness builds as people go beyond simply hoping "*Maybe this group is for me*," "*Maybe I can do this*," and "*Maybe I'm not different*" to the possibility that relating mindfully to psychosis could make a significant difference to their lives.

To strengthen this hope, facilitators listen for and highlight examples of choosing to allow voices, images, thoughts, and other sensations and day-to-day stressors to come and go without reacting. It is also common for people to have moments of *diminished hope* in being able to live with psychosis, perhaps if early optimism gives way to a concern that mindfulness "*isn't working*" or "*isn't going to be enough*." Facilitators validate these moments too, reassuring the group that it is normal when learning mindfulness to have moments of doubt as well as hope, and that these usually ease with practice.

Being Myself More Fully

Understanding and expressing oneself deepens as people learn to describe their experiences of psychosis, often for the first time, and recognize how they relate both reactively and mindfully to these sensations and other stressors. The practice of sharing moments of joy and connection from daily life can feel as exposing as describing psychosis and naming trauma, and also reflects and strengthens people's ability to be themselves. As contributions are consistently met with acceptance and validation, people's willingness to express and be themselves grows, in line with developing universality, cohesion, and hope.

SESSION GUIDANCE

Sessions 3 and 4 Structure

1. Opening the session
2. Review mindfulness practice over the week: reactivity, letting go, formal practice, moments of mindfulness
3. First core mindfulness practice
4. Inquiry focused on first practice

5. *Session 3 psychoeducation:* choosing to let go of habitual distressing reactions by (a) learning to recognize when we are caught in habitual reactivity; (b) recognizing how reactivity feels in the body and mind, and emotionally; and (c) discovering that choice is possible
   Session 4 psychoeducation: choosing to respond mindfully by noticing (a) distressing reactivity, and (b) mindful responding

[Optional break]

6. Second core mindfulness practice
7. Inquiry focused on second practice and session learning points
8. Closing the session and home practice

Handouts/Materials

- Session handout
- Audio recording of core mindfulness practice—for anyone who needs a replacement (either your own recording of the "Core mindfulness practice," or the version we provide online in Track 1; see Appendix 9.1).

Opening the Session

We open sessions by welcoming group members and briefly outlining the structure of the session:

> *"Welcome back, it's good to see everyone. Today is our third/fourth meeting of eight. As usual, we'll do our two mindfulness practices, with some discussion after each. And we'll think about how mindfulness can help us choose how to relate to unpleasant or stressful sensations and situations."*

Check-In on Mindfulness Practice

As in Session 2, opening the session flows into reflective discussion of mindfulness practice since the previous session. For example:

> *"First, it would be good to hear how things went with practicing mindfulness over the last week. How did it go with the recorded practice, and with moments of mindfulness in everyday life?"*

In line with the theme of choice, we briefly explore and contrast any examples of distressing habitual reactivity and mindful responding, and may use these later during inquiry or psychoeducation. At the check-in, we validate and build universality, and probably hold off on guided discovery until later inquiry. We continue to listen for and correct any misunderstandings about mindfulness (e.g., needing to focus on the breath at all times, or not finding mindfulness relaxing). In terms of informal practice, we continue to ask about and validate any moments of mindfulness described: checking in with ourselves, and noticing moments of joy and connection. Additionally, from Session 3, we ask about moments of heightened arousal and stress. We introduce the ABC (awareness, breathing, choice) mnemonic to guide mindful responses in these stressful moments, and include the ABC prompt in the session and handout.

At this stage in the group, we also gently ask anyone who has not spoken about home practice to give some feedback—for example: "*Mo, how did it go for you last week with mindfulness?*" We want to encourage anyone who has yet to listen to the core mindfulness practice at home to give it a try, and consider any barriers—for example: "*Has anyone not yet been able to listen to the 10-minute recording at home?*" (either your own recording of the "Core mindfulness practice," or the version we provide in Track 1 at *www.guilford.com/chadwick-materials*; see Appendix 9.1). If so, we would explore what gets in the way and normalize any difficulty getting started with home practice. For example:

> "*Thanks for sharing that, Grace. Many of us find it easier to practice in a group than alone at home. Is there anything you can think of that might help you try it this week? [Pause] What have others found that helped them practice at home?*"

Guiding the Core Mindfulness Practices

The core mindfulness practice is designed to draw attention to the two-circles model and choice points—that is, how it feels in the body and mind, and emotionally, to be lost in habitual reaction, and how it feels to choose moments of decentered awareness: of stepping back and letting go of reaction, or of the breath and body. At this stage in the group, and prompted by the guidance, people increasingly catch themselves lost in reaction and choose to let this go and return to the sensations of breathing.

Facilitators follow the core mindfulness practice guidance, while allowing themselves the freedom to introduce their own words and to weave in additional phrases to emphasize key points linked to the session theme or from earlier discussion. Some group members feel frustration at still reacting much of the time during mindfulness practice with just a few moments of decentered awareness. Guidance includes phrases that explicitly address frustration and self-criticism, with phrases that encourage kindness, patience, gentleness, and self-acceptance.

- Emphasize we are all doing the best we can—for example, "*as best we can*," "*if we can*"
- Normalize getting lost in reaction and encouraging nonjudgment when this happens—for example, "*If you find you've been lost, there's no need to judge yourself, we all get lost in this way*"
- Convey the importance of gentle concentration—for example, "*It's important not to try too hard to be mindful. If we try too hard, we just make ourselves tense and stressed; see if you can find a level of gentle concentration*"
- Highlight that it is always possible, in this moment, to come back to the breath and begin again—for example, "*When you notice you've been lost in reaction, that's fine, that's just what our minds do—gently bringing your attention back to the breath to begin again*"

The possibility of always being able to come back to the breath and begin again is particularly important for group members who feel frustrated or discouraged. If frustration and self-criticism are strong during inquiry after the first practice, then in the guidance for the second practice it can be helpful to emphasize nonjudgment and patience. For example:

> "*As best you can, let go of judging yourself when you keep getting caught up in reacting to voices, images, thoughts, feelings, and other sensations—this is just what our minds do*" or "*Each time we notice our automatic reactions, we get better at recognizing them—it takes time for us to learn to respond mindfully.*"

In Sessions 3 and 4, we may introduce the idea of silently noting sensations and habitual reactions. This can facilitate decentered awareness by recognizing and stepping back from sensations and reactions. For example:

> "*When you find you have become lost, perhaps just silently noting to yourself where your mind had gone to—maybe 'voices' or 'worries' or 'judging'—and then gently bring your awareness back to your breathing.*"

Facilitating the Two Periods of Inquiry

In all sessions, the first period of inquiry follows and focuses on the first mindfulness practice, and the second follows the second practice, and pulls together key learning from the entire session. From Session 3 onward moments of stepping back and letting go of reactivity are explicitly framed as a *choice*. This is an empowering position, though it needs to be introduced carefully, given how easy it is for people to judge themselves for continuing to get lost in reactivity, causing further distress. Alongside validation, building universality and other group factors, and guiding discovery of metacognitive insights, we remain attentive to the need to embody the qualities of authenticity, acceptance, and trust, and remain watchful for any ongoing misunderstandings about mindfulness.

In these sessions, inquiry is closely linked to the two-circles model and to choosing to allow voices, images, thoughts, and other sensations to come and go without reacting (the middle stage of the core process of change; see Chapter 3). Through guided discovery, we continue to support people to recognize and understand moments of habitual reactivity and mindful responding.

In Sessions 3 and 4, we close the second period of inquiry by inviting each person to share one thing they have learned or that stands out for them from the session. When people are hesitant, we may start with a brief reflection linked to the theme of choice. For example:

> *"I'm struck today by how you all experienced moments of choosing not to react to unpleasant sensations, and how this left you feeling stronger."*

Focusing on Moments of Mindfulness Practice That Support Learning

In Sessions 3 and 4, we continue to listen for comments that illustrate either side of the two-circles model, and guide discovery in an iterative way to support metacognitive understanding about habitual distressing reactions and moments of mindful responding. Additionally, we amplify the choice people have made to respond mindfully, either by stepping back from reactivity, or attending to the sensations of breathing. As well as exploring moments from the core mindfulness practice, we may draw on examples from daily life, prompted by the three informal practices—moments of mindfulness: checking in with ourselves, noticing moments of joy and connection, and stepping back when things are difficult

(ABC). We also emphasize that repeated moments of *choosing to respond mindfully* begin to change a person's relationship with their psychosis.

Attitude Toward Practice

In Sessions 1 and 2 facilitators emphasize a gentle, compassionate approach both to mindfulness practice and the self when learning mindfulness, recognizing that it is hard to step back from unpleasant voices, images, thoughts, feelings, and other sensations. In Sessions 3 and 4 we build on this, reminding group members that mindfulness cannot be forced but requires a gentle, steady commitment, and a willingness to choose to start again and again in the face of frequent setbacks.

Mindfulness is framed as an *additional* way of relating to unpleasant psychosis sensations, thereby avoiding any perceived pressure to abandon familiar, habitual reactions. Facilitators highlight that the aim is to recognize and learn about our patterns of reactivity so we can let these go if we so choose. We draw out the common experience (universality) of being drawn back into instinctive reactivity to unpleasant and frightening sensations; to soften the frustration and self-judgment when this inevitably occurs; and foster the motivation to step back, refocus on our breathing, and begin again and again, no matter how many times we lose present-moment awareness.

Guiding Discovery Related to Habitual Distressing Reactions

In Sessions 1 and 2 we focus on how this feels in the body and mind, and emotionally, to be caught in reactivity. This continues in Sessions 3 and 4, to support all group members to learn to recognize their habitual reactions to unpleasant sensations, and extend this to draw out the impact of *relying exclusively on these habitual reactions.* While we do not expect people to stop reacting (imagine standing calmly in the face of someone screaming abusively), we listen for and highlight any moments when people do step back and let go of habitual reactions, and the choice they have made to do so. Moments of catching oneself reacting are framed as a vital first step in the process of freeing oneself from the tyranny of psychosis.

Drawing Attention to Unhelpful Metacognitive Beliefs

Throughout the group program, facilitators listen for and gently draw attention to unhelpful metacognitive beliefs that maintain habitual reactivity, including linked self-judgments. These are not challenged directly—rather, the effects are explored within the group. In Sessions 3 and 4, we continue with this approach and look for opportunities to draw out helpful metacognitive insights that foster mindful responding. With a growing familiarity with the two-circles model, unhelpful metacognitive beliefs may include versions of "*I should be able to control my mind*"; "*If I let them in, I'll be overwhelmed and lose control*"; and "*I have to keep struggling, keep fighting, or I'll be destroyed.*" Emerging metacognitive insights may include versions of "*Reacting all the time is distressing, exhausting, and leaves me feeling trapped, out of control*"; "*Not reacting is possible, and can feel calming and peaceful*"; and "*I have some choice.*" As group members start to recognize that far from being protective, reactive cycles are *creating* much of their distress, tension, and mental turmoil, they begin to see that there may be an alternative way to alleviate distress and suffering.

Alongside learning that habitual reactions create distress, people begin to see, for themselves and others in the group, that this reactivity is not working (or not working well) in relation to their psychosis. As well as drawing out the impact of reactivity on the person, we draw out the impact on the voices, images, thoughts, feelings, and other sensations, and find that these often become stronger, louder, and more intrusive, leaving people feeling increasingly powerless. Avoidance, struggle, and judgment can give some temporary respite, though this gives the person no opportunity to learn that there may be other, more effective and less distressing ways of coping.

Reevaluating Unhelpful Metacognitive Beliefs: Illustrative Dialogue

As we approach the halfway point of the group program, many people are starting to recognize a version of the unhelpful metacognitive beliefs "*If I let them in, I'll be overwhelmed and lose control*" and "*I have to keep struggling, keep fighting, or I'll be destroyed.*" For others, these remain implicit and as facilitators we listen for *markers* such as imperatives (e.g., "*I must . . . ,*" "*I have to . . . ,*" "*I can't . . .*") and strong emotions, often fear, linked to the suggestion of letting go of familiar, habitual reactions.

Our role is to draw out the (1) belief, (2) feared consequence, and (3) experiential reality of how it actually felt to let go of their reactivity during mindfulness practice. Sometimes this also yields a personalized metacognitive insight. A guided discovery approach enables people to learn that while unhelpful metacognitive beliefs are highly compelling, direct experience during mindfulness practice supports alternative metacognitive insights.

Illustrative dialogue	**Commentary**
FACILITATOR: Gita, I remember you saying last time that even though fighting the voices wasn't working for you, you were worried they'd get worse—stronger, louder—if you didn't fight back.	Facilitator seeks to draw out/clarify unhelpful metacognitive beliefs.
GITA: Yeah. They'd come back full force and then who knows what would happen? I wouldn't know how to cope.	Gita gives feared consequence.
FACILITATOR: Yes, it can feel scary to let go of our usual ways of reacting to difficult experiences; it's a big step. How did it feel during the practice when you let go of resisting and fighting the voices for a few moments?	Facilitator seeks to draw out experiential reality of letting go of reactivity.
GITA: Not so frightening. It's a bit confusing. The voices are always with me, but I'm more aware of where I am, not lost in my own world. I could hear you talking.	Gita describes experiential reality of letting go of reactivity.
FACILITATOR: So, your fear was that if you stopped fighting, you'd feel overwhelmed by the voices. But what actually happened was you felt less scared of the voices and more present, more aware.	Facilitator summarizes to check understanding.
GITA: My mind felt calmer. Felt a bit more in control, you know, I am a little bit more in control. The voices didn't seem so dangerous. There's light at the end of the tunnel—I'm on the right track.	Gita approaches a metacognitive insight: "*When I let go, I have more control.*"

Moments of Mindful Responding

As the program progresses, inquiry focuses increasingly on moments of mindful responding (the right side of the two-circle model), as well as consolidating learning about habitual reactivity (the left side of the model). Facilitators focus on moments of decentered awareness of the breath, body, and psychosis sensations to heighten awareness of how these feel and to draw out learning. We continue to name moments of decentered awareness of voices, images, thoughts, feelings, and other sensations, without reacting, as *moments of mindfulness*.

Facilitators guide discovery of how moments of decentered awareness feel in the body and mind, and emotionally—for example: "*When I heard you say to focus on my breathing, I felt calmer, peaceful for a while,*" and that repeated moments of decentered awareness support the metacognitive insight that "*I can step back and observe voices, images, thoughts, and feelings*" (and the implicit "*Voices, images, and other unpleasant sensations are separate from my reactions to them*"). Facilitators note when individuals have made the choice to allow sensations to come fully into awareness without having to react. As before, just two or three moments of decentered awareness during a 10-minute practice can instill hope and provide a source of metacognitive learning about the impact of sometimes making these choices.

At this stage in the program, many people's reflections and metacognitive insights express spontaneous comparisons between habitual reactivity and mindful responding—for example: "*There's much less fear to it,*" "*It feels safer than I expected,*" and "*Mindfulness is the first time my mind stops moving.*" As facilitators, we note this contrast and the choice made to respond mindfully, and link this back to the two-circles model.

Changing Relationship with Psychosis

For some group members, we see an emerging sense of personal agency. This comes from repeated moments of people catching themselves in reactivity and choosing to step back and let go, or from allowing an unpleasant sensation to come fully into awareness and pass or fade without reacting (*nonreactivity*). As facilitators, we note and name these choice points. This growing awareness of choice and control leads in turn to a shift in the person's relationship with their psychosis:

> "*It seems to me that many of you are finding that you don't always have to fight or struggle with the thoughts, voices, and images. When you step back and choose not to react, it feels calming and empowering. I wonder though, what does this say about the power and control these thoughts, voices, and images have over you?*"

Facilitators guide the group toward the possibility that while we cannot control all that comes into our mind, what comes into our mind does not need to control us! This is an important relational shift for many who joined the group believing that their psychosis ruled their lives.

Common Challenges to Practice at Sessions 3 and 4

Common challenges in Sessions 3 and 4 focus on difficulty recognizing (e.g., "*I don't even notice my mind's wandered*") and letting go of reactivity (e.g., "*I can't let go*"), and frustration and self-criticism for repeatedly getting caught up in habitual reactions (e.g., "*I still can't do this, I'm no good at anything*"). See the following table for common challenges, linked metacognitive beliefs, and possible responses that often arise at this stage in the program. Learning mindfulness is not a linear process, and challenges from Sessions 1 and 2 are likely to persist or recur for many.

Psychoeducation in Sessions 3 and 4

In Sessions 3 and 4, psychoeducation focuses on choosing how to respond to unpleasant sensations. Session 3 focuses on the distress that accompanies reactivity, and the impact of choosing to step back and letting go of these reactions. Session 4 extends this to emphasize how *reactive cycles are creating much of the distress* people feel. While group members learn at their own pace, there is value in facilitators having a clear narrative across sessions, and being able to revisit points when these are likely to benefit individuals.

Session 3 psychoeducation focuses on choosing to let go of habitual distressing reactions by emphasizing three linked aspects of the core process of change in mindfulness for psychosis: (1) learning to recognize when we are caught in habitual reactivity; (2) recognizing how reactivity feels in the body and mind, and emotionally; and (3) discovering that choice is possible.

Learning to Recognize When We Are Caught in Habitual Reactivity

We note that for all of us, it takes practice to recognize our habitual reactions in the moment of experiencing them, and harder still to learn to do so with kindness and letting go of self-judgment. It can be helpful to illustrate this with one or two examples from recent group discussions.

Common Challenges Arising in Sessions 3 and 4, and Possible Responses

Challenges	Examples	Unhelpful metacognitive beliefs and judgments	Possible responses from facilitators
Difficulty noticing and letting go of habitual reactivity	*"I don't even realize what I'm doing, it's just automatic."*	*"I should be able to recognize what I'm doing and stop reacting."*	Build universality and hope. *"It can take time to notice our reactions as they often happen so quickly but it will come with practice."*
	"I can't stop, I have to fight—once I start I can't stop, can't find my way back."	*"If I stop fighting, I'll be overwhelmed; if I don't listen, I'll miss something and it will be worse."*	*"It's very hard to step back and not react to frightening thoughts and images, but what we've seen is that you're already stepping back sometimes, and we can build on this."*
	"I've got to fight back to protect myself, my family."	*"If I stop fighting, worse will come for me and my family."*	Validate and contextualize difficulty. *"So, for a lot of this practice you felt agitated and lost in reacting to fears for yourself and your family, the idea of not fighting is very frightening."* Look for moments of mindfulness; what did the person notice? *"Were there any moments when you noticed the fight in your mind?"*
	"I have to work it out, I have no choice."	*"Until I can work this out, solve it, I'll never be free."*	Guide discovery of metacognitive insights. *"It's understandable you keep trying to work it out if it seems you have no choice, or this is the only way to be free. I wonder, though, what was it like when you did let go for a moment and focused on your breathing?"*
	"If you let them go all the time, what have you got left? Nothing."	*"Letting go of reacting means you lose the sensation."*	Build universality and hope. *"Do others worry about losing their voices? I wonder if letting the voices, thoughts, and feelings come fully into awareness without avoidance and resistance, you'll be able to live your lives more and not less fully."*

Beliefs about being wrong, flawed, bad, useless	*"I can't do this, everyone else can do it, I'm hopeless."*	*"I am fundamentally different and set apart from other people."*	Build universality and hope. *"Well done for bringing your attention to the breath when you could—it's not easy."* *"It's understandable that you got caught up—the images and feelings sound really intrusive and grabbed your attention. It's very common for us all to be swept along by upsetting thoughts or feelings."* To the group: *"Do others find themselves swept away like this?"*
	"I wouldn't have these voices if I wasn't rotten deep down."	*"Bad people have bad thoughts."*	Guide discovery of self-criticism. *"I notice you judged yourself quite harshly there. Is that something you often do? [Pause] How do you feel when you criticize yourself like this?"* To the group: *"So many of us are quick to criticize and judge ourselves, and find it hard to show ourselves the kindness we can show others—how does constant self-criticism and judgment affect us?"*
			Encourage kindness and acceptance. *"Earlier you said you felt OK about not doing any practice last week as things were so stressful at home—you accepted you were doing the best you could. [Pause] What stops us from being kinder, more accepting to ourselves, more of the time?"* *"It seems important for us all to be kinder to ourselves, less self-critical, to accept we are doing our best in very difficult circumstances."*

Recognizing How Reactivity Feels in the Body and Mind, and Emotionally

This too takes time as we are used to these feelings. In the mindfulness practices we prompt people to tune into the distress, physical tension, and mental turmoil that accompany cycles of reactivity. In the subsequent inquiry, we encourage reflection to increase individuals' awareness of the moment-to-moment impact of habitual reactivity.

Discovering That Choice Is Possible

Here, we highlight that people are already sometimes choosing to let go of habitual reactions to psychosis and other stressors, and discuss how this feels, again, in the body and mind, and emotionally. For example:

> *"I'd also like to spend a few minutes talking about choice. We all have unpleasant, frightening, difficult things come into our mind—thoughts, images, voices, feelings. We react quickly to unpleasant experiences, often before we've even thought about how to respond. This is natural as we have evolved to react to signs of threat with avoidance, confrontation, sometimes freezing, and by making quick judgments.*
>
> *"When this comes to threatening experiences in our mind, these quick reactions don't work well, and we get caught up in reactive cycles of avoidance, struggle, and judgment. This brings emotional distress, physical tension, and mental turmoil. The more we get lost in these ways of reacting, the more distressed and exhausted we become. It is possible to ease this distress, this suffering. Although we can't stop unpleasant things coming into our mind, we can choose how we respond.*
>
> *"If we can learn to step back and choose to let go of our usual reactions—respond mindfully—we may feel calmer and stronger. How we respond to unpleasant sensations makes all the difference."*

Session 4 psychoeducation highlights the possibility of choosing to respond mindfully to psychosis and other sensations, using the two-circles model to focus on (1) distressing reactivity and (2) mindful responding.

Distressing Reactivity

Here, we refer explicitly to the two-circles model. We first describe the left side of the model, drawing on people's reflections to illustrate how habitual reactivity—avoidance, struggle, and judgment—are understandable and create distress, physical tension, and mental turmoil. For example:

> *"Over the last two sessions we've seen that we all have unpleasant, frightening, difficult things come into our mind. When this happens, we react instinctively, automatically, and quickly to try to get rid of these voices, images, thoughts, and feelings. We get caught up in avoidance, struggle, and judgments. You are finding that these ways of reacting don't work well for you and often make things worse—creating distress and tension, and leaving you feeling alone with no control or choice. The more we are stuck in these reactive cycles, the worse we feel—reacting all the time makes things worse, not better."*

Mindful Responding

We then outline the right side of the model, to show how stepping back and choosing to respond mindfully reduces distress, tension, and mental turmoil. We suggest that by changing their relationship to psychosis, people may feel more in control of their lives, and have more time and energy to focus on the things that are important to them. For example:

> *"With mindfulness, you are finding that sometimes you can pause, step back, and choose not to react in these automatic ways. And what's so important is that stepping back and choosing to respond mindfully eases distress and tension, and can feel empowering. By doing this, you are starting to change the relationship you have with psychosis. The more you respond mindfully, the more you—not psychosis—are in control of your life."*

Closing the Session, Home Practice, and Handouts

By now, most group members have started to practice mindfulness formally and informally, and we encourage people to continue putting what they are learning into practice over the week, in a way that works for them.

As before, we spend a couple of minutes distributing and describing the session handout. We recommend that anyone who has yet to listen to the audio recording of the core mindfulness practice does so, as this will help them use mindfulness outside the group. In Session 3, we outline a third informal practice:

> *"In addition to the audio recordings, we're encouraging you to practice 'moments of mindfulness.' In the first session, we discussed 'checking in on ourselves'—tuning into sensations in the body and the flow of sensations as we breathe in and breathe out, just for a few moments. In the second session, we encouraged you to notice moments of joy and connection with other people. Please continue with these.*
>
> *"Today we have a third (the last) suggestion for how to practice moments of mindfulness. We'd like you to try this when things are unpleasant or stressful. It's like the great example Hannah shared earlier, when she chose to step back in a stressful situation with her Mom rather than 'explode.' We call it* ABC *to help you remember what to do. It begins with awareness, A. When you are experiencing difficult thoughts, or intrusive voices or images, or are in a stressful situation with someone, just notice that right now things are difficult, stressful. Next is breathing, B. Just as we do in the group when we practice mindfulness, come back to your breathing and draw a couple of natural breaths. Finally, choice,* C. *Ask yourself, 'how do I want to respond right now in this moment?' Awareness, breathing, choice. It's on the handout—I hope you'll try this over the coming week."*

We remind the group that formal and informal home practice is the best way to embed the benefits of mindfulness in daily life, and encourage people to record any observations, reflections, and questions on the handouts. Around this point in the program, many people are spontaneously reporting making valued behavioral changes, and we encourage this in our closing remarks, perhaps saying "And finally, do keep looking for opportunities to find more meaning and connection in your daily lives, taking small steps that feel important and meaningful to you." We then close the session with warm wishes for the week to come—for example: *"Thank you for coming today. We hope you all have a good week and look forward to seeing each of you next time."*

Mindfulness Group: Session 3 Handout

Reacting to Unpleasant Sensations

We all react to unpleasant sensations quickly and instinctively—we try to avoid or escape, we resist, struggle, or freeze, and we often make quick judgments. These are natural reactions but they usually make difficult voices, images, thoughts, and feelings even stronger, and leave us distressed and exhausted.

Mindfulness Brings Choice: We Don't Always Have to React in These Ways

By practicing mindfulness, we learn how to pause and step back from difficult voices, images, thoughts, and feelings. With practice, this gives us a choice: whether to react in the usual automatic ways or slow down and respond mindfully. When we can step back and allow difficult experiences to come into awareness and then pass or fade without getting lost in reactivity, we feel calmer, stronger.

Please make a note of one or two things you learned in Session 3:

____

____

____

____

____

____

____

____

There may be many times this week when you get caught up in instinctive and habitual reactions to difficult voices, images, thoughts, and feelings. As best you can, remind yourself that you are only just starting to learn mindfulness and doing the best you can—it takes time to learn to respond differently to unpleasant and stressful experiences.

(continued)

From *Mindfulness for Psychosis: A Group Therapy Approach*, by Paul Chadwick, Katherine Newman-Taylor, and Nicola Abba. Copyright © 2027 The Guilford Press. Permission to photocopy this material, or to download and print enlarged versions (*www.guilford.com/chadwick-materials*), is granted to purchasers of this book for personal use or use with clients; see copyright page for details.

Home Practice

This week, as best you can:

- *Practice guided mindfulness*—listen to the 10-minute audio recording; try to listen at least 2 or 3 times this week.
- *Notice moments of mindfulness*—"checking in with ourselves" (tuning into the sensations of breathing), noticing moments of joy and connection, and practicing ABC (awareness, breathing, choice)

Stepping Back When Things Are Difficult: ABC

When you are experiencing unpleasant voices, images, thoughts, or feelings, or when you are in a stressful situation, use ABC to take a moment of mindfulness:

- *Awareness*—pause, step back, and just notice that things right now are difficult, stressful
- *Breathing*—come back to your breathing and take a few natural breaths
- *Choice*—ask yourself, "How do I want to respond right now in this moment?"

Week 3 Diary

Over the week, jot down anything you notice or learn from practicing mindfulness between sessions. You may wish to share your reflections with the group in the next session:

Mindfulness Group: Session 4 Handout

Today we talked about the possibility of *choosing* how to respond to unpleasant sensations. This can be hard when we've used other ways of coping, often for many years.

The Two-Circles Model:
Distressing Reaction and Mindful Responding

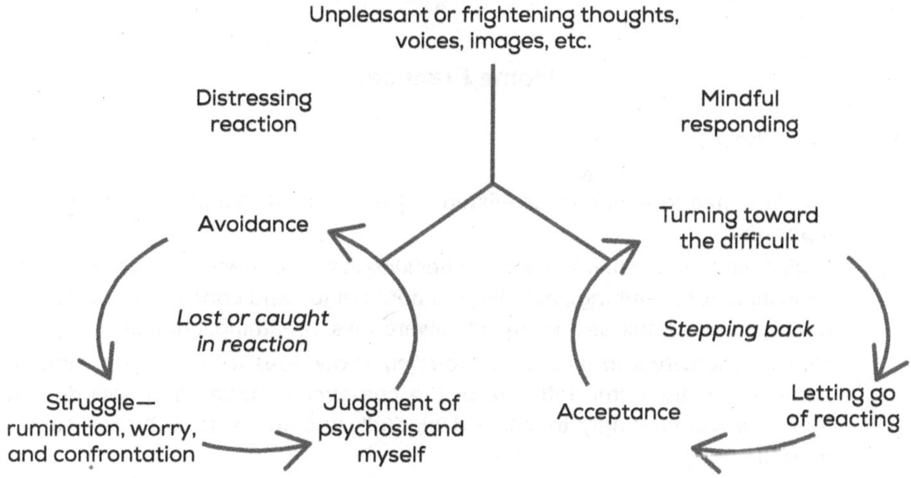

When unpleasant sensations come into awareness, we often become lost in reaction—we try to avoid or get rid of these experiences, struggle with rumination, worry, and confrontation, and are quick to make judgments. These ways of reacting are understandable but create distress, tension, and exhaustion.

Mindfulness is a different way of responding—allowing difficult experiences to come into awareness and then pass or fade, without avoiding, struggling, or judging psychosis or ourselves. For all of us, unpleasant, frightening, and disturbing sensations come into our mind, and while we cannot control all that comes into our mind, we can decide how we respond. When we choose not to react, we often feel calmer, stronger, and more in control of our lives.

(continued)

From *Mindfulness for Psychosis: A Group Therapy Approach*, by Paul Chadwick, Katherine Newman-Taylor, and Nicola Abba. Copyright © 2027 The Guilford Press. Permission to photocopy this material, or to download and print enlarged versions (*www.guilford.com/chadwick-materials*), is granted to purchasers of this book for personal use or use with clients; see copyright page for details.

Please make a note of one or two things you learned in Session 4:

____

____

____

____

Home Practice

This week, as best you can:

- *Practice guided mindfulness*—listen to the 10-minute audio recording, daily if possible
- *Notice moments of mindfulness*—"checking in with ourselves" (tuning into the sensations of breathing), noticing moments of joy and connection, and stepping back when things are difficult (awareness, breathing, choice)
- *Notice reactivity and mindful responding*—how does it feel to be caught in habitual reactivity (the left side of the two-circles model) and how does it feel, however fleetingly, to respond mindfully (the right side of the two-circles model)?

Week 4 Diary

Over the week, jot down anything you notice or learn from practicing mindfulness between sessions. You may wish to share your reflections with the group in the next session:

____

____

____

____

____

____

____

____

11

Sessions 5 and 6: Accepting Psychosis and Myself

The theme for Sessions 5 and 6 is *acceptance*. By this point in the program, most group members are showing one another kindness and acceptance. Some are also starting (hesitantly, intermittently) to show some acceptance of their own experiences of psychosis and of themselves. This develops through mindfulness practice; facilitators' modeling of acceptance, trust, and authenticity; and the growing sense of universality and other group factors. For many, judging psychosis and themselves is a deeply ingrained habit. As facilitators, we recognize that acceptance is an ongoing and challenging process, and validate moments of acceptance when these arise, however fleetingly.

We introduce the idea of acceptance carefully. The invitation is *to accept that psychosis sensations, stripped of emotional distress, physical tension, and mental turmoil, are happening.* For people who have believed, often for many years, that they have to fight voices, images, and perceived persecutors to survive, the possibility of acceptance is supported by a growing awareness of choice and control in how to relate to these sensations, and the sense of empowerment this brings.

Facilitators emphasize that we all experience unpleasant sensations, that this is part of being human, but that these experiences do not define us. Accepting psychosis and accepting the self are therefore closely related psychological processes. In group sessions, we foster acceptance that psychosis sensations are occurring, and encourage nonreactivity. In this way, psychosis becomes less and less the basis for self-definition, allowing acceptance of the self to emerge—the possibility of accepting oneself as someone who experiences psychosis.

Facilitating Group Factors in Sessions 5 and 6

In the second half of the program, facilitators often notice an important shift in focus, with group members spontaneously talking less about psychosis and more about their daily lives, relationships, and hopes for the future. We embrace this wider focus, while continuing to reflect on the costs of reactivity, and guide discovery of metacognitive insights about psychosis and sources of distress and well-being.

Universality

In the initial sessions, universality is founded on recognizing that others have similar problems and struggles. In Sessions 3 and 4, this extends to a shared understanding of how it feels in the body and mind, and emotionally, to respond mindfully to psychosis and more broadly to moments of joy and connection. In Sessions 5 and 6, for some group members, universality extends further to be more *person based* than *experience based* through an emerging metacognitive insight that "*I am a person like others*"—a recognition of shared humanity. This is a profound, though initially fragile, change. When this happens, we tread carefully, aware of the sense of difference, of being set apart and less than human, that dominates the lives of many people with psychosis. We look for opportunities to reflect and reinforce this shift—for example: "*From our conversation today, it sounds like you are discovering you have a lot in common as people,*" or "*It's good to hear you're finding that living with psychosis is just one thing you have in common.*"

Cohesion

At this stage in the group program, psychological safety, trust, and connection within the group are usually well established. Fears about being judged or viewed as different are often largely absent. Moments of connection are experienced and enjoyed in the group as well as between sessions in people's daily lives. Group members may use spontaneous humor and facilitators may also feel more comfortable using humor. Facilitators look for opportunities to convey their trust in the group, perhaps acknowledging their own uncertainty about a discussion point and seeking the group's advice and feedback. Facilitators continue to listen for and validate expressions of kindness among group members. As cohesion grows, concerns about the program ending emerge: the loss of the group and worries about maintaining progress without this support. We acknowledge these concerns and confirm that we will discuss the group ending, as well as practical next steps, in some detail in the final sessions.

Hope

A growing sense of agency accompanies a recognition of the choice and control people have over how they relate to psychosis sensations and start to "*Reclaim my power through acceptance*" (see Chapter 3). With agency comes hope for personal recovery as people discover how responding mindfully enhances mental and physical well-being. Previously, hope rested on finding a way to defeat unpleasant voices, images, thoughts, and feelings; now hope focuses on learning to live well with psychosis. This arises from acceptance that these sensations are occurring and finding the courage and persistence to respond mindfully, and so free themselves from the tyranny of psychosis and dehumanization of the self. People recognize (and we confirm) that sustaining this will be challenging, and for all of us, the ability to respond mindfully ebbs and flows. We gently guard against hopes being raised too high too soon, balancing this by recognizing the shift from an external to an internal locus of control, and affirm people's emerging self-confidence and optimism about the future.

Being Myself More Fully

In the second half of the program, many people start to see psychosis as "*Part of who I am*" rather than defining who they are. This "*Knowing I am more than psychosis*" reinforces an acceptance that these sensations are occurring and allows people to express other aspects of themselves in the group. As facilitators, we listen for and validate such comments. We may also describe how we too can struggle to be ourselves—for example: "*I still get a little anxious sometimes about expressing myself, maybe in a meeting at work, but that's OK; being ourselves with other people can take time.*" To normalize the ongoing process of being oneself, we seek to ease group members' anxieties about expressing themselves more fully and support self-acceptance.

SESSION GUIDANCE

Sessions 5 and 6 Structure

1. Opening the session
2. Review mindfulness practice over the week—habitual reactivity and mindful responding through formal practice and moments of mindfulness
3. First core mindfulness practice
4. Inquiry focused on first practice
5. *Session 5 psychoeducation:* accepting psychosis sensations, stripped of reactions, and recognizing we all experience unpleasant sensations

   Session 6 psychoeducation: accepting ourselves, focusing on (a) knowing I am more than the psychosis and (b) recognizing I am fundamentally the same as other people

[Optional break]

6. Second core mindfulness practice
7. Inquiry focused on second practice and session learning points
8. Closing the session and home practice

Handouts

- Session handout

Opening the Session

As before, we start by warmly welcoming group members and outlining the plan for the session. We also note the session number and how many remain. For example:

> *"Good to see you all. This is our fifth/sixth meeting of eight. As usual, we'll do two mindfulness practices together and discuss what you can take from these. Today, we'd also like to talk about the importance of acceptance."*

Check-In on Mindfulness Practice

After opening the session, we seek feedback on mindfulness practice over the week. This includes the core mindfulness practice (either your own recording or the version we provide online in Track 1; see Appendix 9.1) and all three informal practices (*moments of mindfulness*): checking in with ourselves (e.g., in neutral moments), noticing moments of joy and connection, and the ABC prompt (e.g., when things are unpleasant or stressful). We listen for understanding of the practices, barriers, and facilitators to regular use, and beneficial effects. We remind the group how these practices collectively embed mindfulness in daily life. Group members often begin to spontaneously share how being in the group is leading them to take steps toward recovery, such as visiting a coffee shop or contacting a friend of family member. We welcome and encourage these behavioral changes and link them to growing mindfulness and self-acceptance in daily life.

As group factors strengthen and people become more comfortable talking together, facilitators may need to contain the check-in part of the session more actively, to keep to the time frame. We are conscious of who usually speaks more and less, and try to offer time to all. At the start of the session, we prioritize validation and building universality. Where opportunities arise for guided discovery of metacognitive beliefs and insights, we keep these in mind for later discussion. For example:

> *"It's great to hear your reflections and we'll continue to discuss these later. We want to make sure we fit in our two practices and have time to discuss these too. Let's do our first practice now."*

In Session 6, if not raised spontaneously in the feedback, we ask about acceptance and judging. For example:

> *"Last week we talked about acceptance and allowing difficult voices, images, thoughts, and feelings to come and go, without getting caught up in judgments. Did anyone notice any moments when they were able to step back and choose not to get caught up in judging the voices, images, thoughts, or themselves? [Pause] How did this feel—in your body and mind, and emotionally—to let go of judging for a few moments?"*

Guiding the Core Mindfulness Practices

In the first half of the program, we tend not to talk about *accepting* unpleasant voices, images, thoughts, feelings, or other sensations, because this can be easily misunderstood and feel invalidating. To this point, the guidance describes *allowing* sensations to come into awareness and pass or fade, which conveys a similar meaning and is less likely to be misunderstood. From Session 5 (second practice), we adapt the core mindfulness practice to draw attention to the impact of habitual judging and self-criticism, and to introduce the term *acceptance*. For example:

> "*Often, we find we've been lost, maybe struggling with voices, caught up in rumination, worry or judgments, and self-criticism. As best you can, notice how it feels to be caught up in judgment and self-criticism, and then how it feels to let this go and reconnect with the next in-breath. We all get lost like this.*
>
> "*Whatever is present in your mind right now, there's no need for judgment. Accepting in this moment—this is my experience—and noticing how this feels in the body, and emotionally, is to accept rather than struggle with these sensations.*
>
> "*For the last minute, as best we can, really being open to and accepting whatever sensations arise, whether pleasant or unpleasant or neutral.*"

We encourage silent noting sparingly. Noting can help people to decenter during practice from psychosis experience (e.g., by silently noting "*voices*," or "*images*") and habitual reactivity (e.g., by silently noting "*struggle*," "*worry*," or "*judgments*"). Occasionally, it can be helpful to go beyond this and encourage a person also to note the *unpleasantness* of the experience too—for example, noting "*unpleasant image*," or "*unpleasant thoughts*." This can be particularly helpful for people who struggle not to get caught up in judging psychosis sensations.

Simon experienced voices and images that he found obscene and highly distressing. He believed he needed to react forcefully: "*When I react, I react strongly. It's a bad thought. It needs to be corrected or put right. The struggle is everything.*" Simon found it helpful to silently note the unpleasantness of the sensation and separate this from his reaction—for example: "*As best you can, silently note 'unpleasant image' or 'unpleasant thought' [pause] and silently note any reactivity—struggle, judgment.*" During inquiry we can clarify that *unpleasant* describes the emotional tone of the sensation (see Chapter 2), and the judgment is what we bring to the sensation (e.g., obscene).

Facilitating the Two Periods of Inquiry

Acceptance of unpleasant psychosis sensations and self-acceptance are closely related processes. The corollary is also true: that habitual judgment of unpleasant sensations and habitual judgment of the self are mutually reinforcing. Judging voices, images, thoughts, feelings, and other sensations is therefore a serious threat to self-acceptance because it leads easily to criticism of the self through unhelpful metacognitive beliefs such as "*Our thoughts and voices reveal who we really are*" and "*Bad people have bad thoughts.*" When people start to let go of judging psychosis sensations, judgment of themselves also lessens. As Sally put it: "*If I'm judging the thoughts I have, I can judge myself as good or bad. If I'm not judging, it makes me feel better about myself.*" For this reason, while Session 5 focuses on accepting psychosis sensations, and Session 6 on self-acceptance, inquiry often addresses both.

A growing acceptance of psychosis is reflected in people's *felt sense* of decentering from these sensations and articulated as metacognitive insights. Decentered awareness of sensations (the right side of the two-circles model; see Chapter 2, Figure 2.1) involves choosing to step back and allow voices, images, thoughts, feelings, and other sensations to come fully into awareness and then pass or fade without avoidance, struggle, or judgment. For many people in the group, moments of acceptance occur more frequently now but are likely to be cut short by familiar intrusive voices, images, and habitual self-judgments. The invitation to step back and begin again and again remains essential throughout the program.

Accepting psychosis is a recognition that in this moment, this is my experience, an understanding that I cannot prevent this, a willingness to open awareness to include sensations as they arise, and the felt sense of doing so. This can be captured (in language) as metacognitive insights about the nature of psychosis and the self—for example: "*We all have unpleasant thoughts, feelings, and sensations*"; "*I cannot control the psychosis and it does not have to control me*"; "*When I accept my psychosis and myself, I feel more human*"; "*I am fundamentally the same as other people*"; and "*I am more than my psychosis.*"

Throughout inquiry, we take opportunities to clarify the meaning of acceptance and address any misunderstandings. For example:

> "*As a reminder, accepting unpleasant voices, images, thoughts, or feelings does not mean that we agree with them, or that we like or want them,*

nor does it mean we give in to them. Accepting is recognizing—Right now, this is my experience and I cannot stop these thoughts and voices coming into my mind; the best thing I can do is to step back, take a breath, allow it to come into awareness, and then pass or fade without struggle, without judgment."

Facilitators continue to draw on the two-circles model and highlight choice in deciding how to relate to unpleasant sensations, as needed. As usual, we close the second period of inquiry by inviting people to share something they have learned or that stands out from the session, and may include a reflection of our own. For example:

"I hear that for each of you, there are some moments when you accept that voices, images, fears, or confusion are present and can let them come and go, and that in these moments, you feel calmer, more yourselves, that you are more than these experiences; they do not define who you are."

Focusing on Moments of Mindfulness Practice That Support Learning

Facilitators continue to focus on moments from the mindfulness practice that illustrate habitual reactivity or mindful responding, guiding people's attention to the felt sense of decentering from unpleasant sensations and habitual reactivity, and discovery of linked metacognitive insights, particularly regarding judgment and acceptance. We note how repeated moments of choosing to respond mindfully support self-acceptance as well as a more empowered relationship with psychosis.

Facilitators attend to moments of mindful responding and support people to articulate linked metacognitive insights when these arise. Importantly, we do not force this, and do not need to draw out all metacognitive insights implicit in inquiry. Rather, we lean into the attitudinal quality of trust—we trust the core process of change, focus discussion on key moments of practice, and trust that people will articulate their experiential learning themselves when ready to do so.

Attitude toward Practice

As in previous sessions, we model and encourage a gentle, compassionate approach to mindfulness practice and to ourselves when learning mindfulness. We emphasize that acceptance is not a task to be completed but an ongoing process of meeting difficult sensations mindfully again and again. This is a big ask, as described by Laura: "*When I find it hard to accept them is when I wake in the morning and they are there, straightaway. A person has a right to some peace, some quiet in this world.*" Facilitators validate the challenge of repeatedly accepting persistent, unpleasant psychosis sensations, and build universality about the inevitable ebb and flow of acceptance. As the program progresses, we also reflect on how acceptance deepens with regular mindfulness practice and time, and that periods of reactivity often become briefer and less intense—people do not go back to square one.

Guiding Discovery Related to Habitual Distressing Reactions and Helpful Metacognitive Insights

Guided discovery continues to focus on recognizing how it feels in the body and mind, and emotionally, to be caught in reactivity. In Sessions 5 and 6 this focuses on understanding the impact of habitual judgment and self-criticism, even self-hatred. Again, we clarify that we are not expecting people immediately to stop judging unpleasant psychosis sensations or themselves but to learn to recognize these habitual cycles of judgment, and notice how it feels to sometimes choose to step back and let go of judging. We consolidate the metacognitive insight that "*Judging creates distress, tension, exhaustion, and mental turmoil.*"

Acceptance is sometimes understood by facilitators to mean a letting go of all judgments. In mindfulness for psychosis groups, we do not necessarily target *initial, automatic judgments*, but focus on the *repetitive judgments triggered* by initial appraisals, which create the greatest suffering. To illustrate, Usha, a new mother, heard voices when bathing her baby daughter, shouting "*drown it, drown it, drown it*" and saw highly distressing images linked to these voices. She steadfastly described the voices and images as "*bad and horrible.*" In the mindfulness group, we did not encourage Usha to let go of this judgment (which would be confusing with little to be gained). Instead, we supported her to learn to step back before this initial, automatic judgment triggered cycles of repetitive and distressing judgments about her failure as a mother and self-hatred ("*What kind of mother has this in her head? There's something really wrong with me*"). Usha learned silently to label these as *unpleasant voices and images* during practice, significantly easing her distress.

Moments of catching oneself lost in judging, as with all habitual reactions, are normalized and framed as opportunities to learn to recognize the impact of reactivity. Inquiry draws attention to the impact of repetitive judgment, self-criticism, and even self-dehumanization:

> *"It's been striking today how quickly many of you get caught in self-criticism and even self-hatred, and how voices can reinforce this. I wonder, how does this affect you? How does this affect your self-esteem, how you live your lives, how you see yourselves?"*

Drawing Attention to Unhelpful Metacognitive Beliefs

We continue to draw out unhelpful metacognitive beliefs that maintain distressing reactivity, with increasing emphasis on judgment and acceptance. These beliefs can then be contrasted with people's direct experience of stepping back and letting go of judgment and any moments of acceptance. We look for opportunities to emphasize choice in how to relate to psychosis sensations and the self, and the impact of choosing to respond mindfully—to psychosis and the self—with greater kindness and acceptance.

Framing Moments of Mindful Responding as Acceptance

Facilitators now start to use moments of mindful responding and moments of acceptance interchangeably. Accepting unpleasant sensations becomes possible when stripped of the distress, tension, and mental turmoil that accompanies habitual reactivity. We prompt people to identify such moments, and draw out how these feel:

> *"Were there any moments when you were able to accept the voice, image, or thought? Allowing the sensation to be there for longer than usual, without turning your attention away or reacting? How did this feel—in your body and mind, and emotionally?"*

Likewise, we draw out how it feels to catch oneself judging and choose to step back and let this go:

> *"Any moments when you noticed you were judging—the images or fears for being there, or yourself for having them—and were then able to choose to step back and let go of judging? How did this feel—in your body and mind, and emotionally?"*

In this way, we guide people to recognize judging as a reaction, and we can choose to let go of judging just as we can let go of pushing difficult sensations away, or becoming caught up in struggle. By drawing out the contrasting effects of judgment and acceptance, people learn versions of the metacognitive beliefs: "*When I let go of judging, I feel calmer, stronger, more in control*"; "*I cannot control the psychosis and it does not have to control me*"; "*When I accept my psychosis and myself, I feel more human*"; and "*I am more than my psychosis.*"

The notion of self-acceptance is often hard for people who have survived living with psychosis with struggle and judgment for many years. We do not directly challenge beliefs about the need to react in these ways but gently draw people's attention to the effects of repetitive self-criticism, to the person's qualities that do not fit with these beliefs, and to the impact of moments of acceptance. As noted above, we do not necessarily target initial, automatic judgments but focus on the repetitive judgments triggered by initial appraisals that create suffering, framing habitual self-criticism and dehumanization as a learned mental habit that diminishes the person's sense of self and holds them back in their daily lives.

Through practicing mindfulness, repeatedly choosing to respond mindfully rather than reactively, and hearing others' accounts of struggling with psychosis and judging themselves, group members become more accepting of themselves, and hopeful about the possibility of personal recovery. As Neil put it:

> "*I would judge me on my thoughts, my voices, my images . . . listening to someone else's experience, who I regard as so-called normal, or whatever, and that their experience was the same, that helped me accept a big chunk about myself. I've thought that basically that I'm not wrong, that I'm quite acceptable.*"

Accepting Psychosis Sensations and the Self—Illustrative Quotes

As facilitators, we listen for and validate acceptance of psychosis sensations and the self. People express a growing acceptance in different ways. For example:

> "*The rush of thoughts came just now but I didn't push them away straightaway. They came in and I went 'OK, here we go,' and I was back to my breathing. It was a bit scary, but they went. And then they came again*

and I did the same thing. And later they came again, and I just did the same. I just didn't react—I didn't know I could do that."—SHALINA

"*You don't lose your mind to them.*"—MARTIN

"*When they come, don't stop them or run away with them. Just accept they're there, give it a little time, you know, like a small child who's got themselves into a state—stay calm, try not to overreact, it will pass.*"
—GREG

"*The instinct is to push them away, send them away. The problem is it never works. Acceptance is essential—you have to accept that you can't do what you instinctively want to do. It's having faith that they will go even if you don't push them away.*"—KAITLIN

"*You don't have to worry about what's right and what's wrong in your head, you know; it's that not judging what's going through your head, it's just accepting it as what it is, not worried about vindictive voices, or whatever, it's just accepting it, that's the way it is. No right, no wrong.*"
—NEIL

"*You know this big thing that comes in with lots of bluster, if you do that it will deflate down, and deflate to this tiny little thing you can just discard. You know it's just a load of hot air and bluster.*"—STEVE

"*Let the voices happen and you'll find out they meant nothing anyway. How can I put it? If you've got voices controlling you, try and just let it and then you'll find out that it didn't control you after all. It's just a voice.*"—GARETH

"*Acceptance that perhaps that I'm no different . . . that I'm no different from anybody else and the acceptance of it, that . . . that's the way it was for other people as well, that was a big one.*"—NEIL

Common Challenges to Practice at Sessions 5 and 6

Common challenges arising in Sessions 5 and 6 typically focus on people's aversion to accepting the presence of psychosis sensations, and difficulty in accepting themselves without judgments that have calcified over many years. Before the session, we also encourage facilitators to review challenges that commonly arise in earlier sessions, which persist or recur for many. See the following table for common challenges and possible responses that may arise at this stage.

When people start to accept psychosis sensations, this results in a step change in their relationship both with their psychosis and themselves.

Psychoeducation in Sessions 5 and 6

In line with the theme for these sessions, the focus of psychoeducation is acceptance. Stepping back, turning toward the difficult, choosing to let go of habitual reactivity, and acceptance of internal sensations and the self, are inseparable facets of mindful responding. In each of the psychoeducation sections of Sessions 1–6, we focus on one aspect of mindful responding, in a sequence that reflects the core process of change. Acceptance builds on the direct experience of stepping back and choosing to let go of familiar reactions, and the direct experience of universality within the group. As always, psychoeducation takes a conversational tone, and facilitators draw on illustrative examples from the session.

Session 5 psychoeducation focuses on accepting the presence of unpleasant sensations, emphasizing (1) that we all experience unpleasant, frightening, and disturbing thoughts, images, and other sensations; and (2) acceptance of psychosis sensations.

We all Experience Unpleasant, Frightening, and Disturbing Thoughts, Images, and Other Sensations

This is not to underestimate the often-devastating impact of psychosis. The intention here is to highlight the universality (and therefore fundamentally human quality) of unwanted intrusions, and crucially, that *we cannot stop this from happening.* If it were possible to get rid of or defeat these sensations, people with psychosis, many of whom live with arguably the most intrusive, disturbing, and overwhelming mental intrusions, would have found a way to do so. While medication is useful for some, this does not work or work sufficiently for many, and the side effects are intolerable to others.

Acceptance of Psychosis Sensations

Acceptance of psychosis sensations involves allowing these sensations to come into awareness and pass or fade without getting caught up in

Common Challenges Arising in Sessions 5 and 6, and Possible Responses

Challenges	Examples	Unhelpful metacognitive beliefs and judgments	Possible responses from facilitators
Difficulty accepting psychosis sensations	*"It's too much to ask of anyone to live with this."*	*"It's wrong to think these things."*	Look for moments of mindfulness. *"Were there any moments when you felt more accepting of the fears that come to your mind? How did you feel in those moments?"*
	"I can't bear it—I didn't ask for this, and I don't want them, it's wrong."	*"I can't bear this."*	Build universality and hope. *"It is hard. One thing I find helpful is to take very small steps. I remind myself—I have had moments of accepting that very upsetting thoughts come into my mind, so I can have more of these moments. Perhaps not right now, but perhaps in the next practice, or tomorrow."*
	"I can only survive if I get rid of them."	*"I have to keep fighting, or I'll be overwhelmed."*	Guide discovery of metacognitive insights. *"When you get lost in fighting and judging, how do you feel? [Pause] So you feel bad and start to beat yourself up for having the voices. And when you mentioned last week that you were able to step back from the fight, just briefly, and focus on your breath, how did this feel?".* *"What we've seen in the group is that we all have unpleasant sensations—whether voices, images, thoughts, or feelings. This is how humans are. We all sometimes have unpleasant, frightening, disturbing things come into our mind. What do others make of the fact that we all have these experiences?"*

Difficulty accepting oneself	*"If I think it, I must want it—it shows I'm wicked."*	*"Our thoughts and voices reveal who we really are."*	Validate and build universality. *"It's so easy for us to think we are different, there's something wrong with us, and that's why we have these experiences. Yet we all have unpleasant thoughts, images, memories, or voices. These are just a part of being human. They don't define us. We are much more than this."*
	"Only someone evil hears evil voices."	*"Bad people have bad thoughts."*	Guide discovery of metacognitive insights. *"It sounds like this habit of judging yourself is creating much of the distress you're finding hard to bear. How does it feel when you step back and accept they are there, not get caught up in judging yourself?"* *"So, you noticed you were judging and hating yourself, and then you were able to step back, let go, and come back to your breathing. How does it feel when you let go of judging yourself?"*
	"People shouldn't see these things—there's something very wrong with me."	*"I am fundamentally different and set apart from other people."*	Validate the impact of self-judgment. *"So, these harsh judgments feel really punishing. You already have troubling thoughts and memories in your head, and on top of this are all these judgments and self-criticism that make you feel even worse."*
			Build self-compassion and kindness. *"What stops us being kinder to ourselves, more self-compassionate?"* *"What helps us be kinder to ourselves, and less judgmental?"* *"What would it be like to let go of these judgments, even for a few moments—to notice the voices and thoughts, and choose to step back rather than joining in with them? How might that feel?"* *"So, when you are mindful, you feel more human."*

reactions that, while completely understandable, inevitably create distress, tension, and mental turmoil. When these sensations dominate and take center stage, the invitation is to allow them to come fully into awareness. When these pass or fade, returning to the background, we return our attention to the sensations of breathing. In this way, the raw sensations—of voices, images, automatic thoughts, memories, feelings, and so on—stripped of distressing reactivity, may be accepted moment-to-moment. Combining the point that we all experience unpleasant sensations, and the possibility of accepting psychosis sensations, we might say:

> *"Today, we'd like to talk more about acceptance. Acceptance is at the heart of mindfulness, and a key part of the two-circles model. What does accepting unpleasant voices, images, thoughts, and memories mean? It does not mean we agree, want, or approve of these voices, images, thoughts, and memories, or will give in to them. When we talk about acceptance in this group, we mean (1) recognizing that we can't stop unpleasant sensations from coming into our mind; (2) stepping back and allowing these sensations to come fully into awareness and pass or fade without reacting in ways that are understandable but create distress—avoiding, struggling, judging; (3) we mean knowing that these are just part of our lives, part of who we are—we experience them, but they do not define us; and (4) acceptance means learning to be kinder, more compassionate to ourselves rather than judging ourselves for having these experiences. People who learn to accept these experiences start to feel more in control of their lives."*

Session 6 psychoeducation focuses on accepting the self by (1) knowing I am more than the psychosis and (2) recognizing I am fundamentally the same as other people.

Knowing I Am More Than the Psychosis

This metacognitive insight emerges toward the end of the mindfulness group program, typically for those who have had repeated experiences of accepting psychosis sensations through regular practice:

> *"Last time we talked about accepting unpleasant voices, thoughts, and other experiences. Today we want to talk about self-acceptance. This begins with the recognition that we all have unpleasant, frightening, and disturbing thoughts, memories, images, and other experiences. For*

some people, including all of you here in this group, these sensations are extreme, overwhelming at times. Self-acceptance means letting go of judging and criticizing yourselves for having these experiences, and choosing to be kinder to yourself, recognizing that you are so much more than the psychosis experiences."

Recognizing I Am Fundamentally the Same as Other People

This linked metacognitive insight describes a depth of understanding of universality. Like other learning in mindfulness groups, this ebbs and flows for group members. This might be introduced as:

> *"Unwanted and disturbing sensations are part of being human and don't set you apart, don't make you different from other people. Many of us are quick to judge and criticize ourselves. We have heard in the group how strong this self-criticism can become, and how living with psychosis can lead you to feel different and set apart from other people, that you have less value, and even are less human. Self-acceptance means knowing that you are not different, that we are all alike, with a shared common humanity. Accepting ourselves in this way empowers us to be ourselves more fully and determine how we want to live our lives."*

Closing the Session, Home Practice, and Handouts

In Sessions 5 and 6, we suggest people attend to moments of judging and moments of acceptance when practicing mindfulness, both formally and informally. Distributing and describing the session handouts gives an opportunity to ask about the three ways to practice informally (and rehearse these if needed), and encourage people to write down any reflections or questions following home practice for the next session.

At this stage in the program, it is helpful to remind people of (1) the importance of the core mindfulness practice (either your own recording of the "Core mindfulness practice," or the version we provide online in Track 1; see Appendix 9.1) as the main way to embed mindfulness in their daily life, and (2) the previous handouts that can be reviewed to strengthen understanding of mindfulness for psychosis.

Finally, we encourage everyone to practice what they are learning in a way that works for them, and offer warm wishes for the week ahead.

Mindfulness Group: Session 5 Handout

Acceptance

Acceptance is at the heart of mindfulness. Accepting difficult voices, images, thoughts, and feelings *does not mean we agree, want, or approve of them, or will give in to them.*

In mindfulness for psychosis groups, acceptance means:

- Recognizing we can't stop unpleasant sensations coming into our mind
- Stepping back and allowing difficult sensations to come into awareness and pass or fade without reacting in ways that create distress—avoiding, struggling, judging
- Knowing these are just part of our lives, part of who we are, and do not define us
- Being kinder and compassionate rather than judging ourselves for having these unpleasant experiences

Accepting difficult experiences without being overwhelmed by them is empowering and helps us feel more in control of our emotions and our mind.

Judging

The opposite of acceptance is judging. This is an understandable reaction—for example, we have a thought and we judge it to be a *bad thought*, then maybe judge ourselves for having it if we believe *bad people have bad thoughts*. Judging creates suffering—it is not part of the experience itself, and we can learn to let go of judgment.

Accepting difficult voices, images, thoughts, and feelings isn't something we do just once. We need to keep doing this again and again. This is easier sometimes than at other times. We need to learn to be kind to ourselves, and not judge our judging!

Please make a note of one or two things you learned in Session 5:

____

____

____

(continued)

From *Mindfulness for Psychosis: A Group Therapy Approach*, by Paul Chadwick, Katherine Newman-Taylor, and Nicola Abba. Copyright © 2027 The Guilford Press. Permission to photocopy this material, or to download and print enlarged versions (*www.guilford.com/chadwick-materials*), is granted to purchasers of this book for personal use or use with clients; see copyright page for details.

Home Practice

This week, as best you can:

- *Notice judging*—of your experiences and yourself
- *Notice acceptance*—of any moments when you can let these judgments go, accepting, in this moment, that this is my experience right now, and notice how this feels
- *Practice guided mindfulness*—listen to the 10-minute audio recording, daily if possible
- *Notice moments of mindfulness*—"checking in with ourselves" (tuning into the sensations of breathing, anytime, anywhere), noticing moments of joy and connection (what are these for you?), and stepping back when things are stressful, using the ABC (*awareness*—of what's happening right now, *breathing*—take a few natural breaths, *choice*—how do you want to respond right now in this moment?)

Week 5 Diary

Over the week, jot down anything you notice or learn from practicing mindfulness between sessions. You may wish to share your reflections with the group in the next session:

Mindfulness Group: Session 6 Handout

Self-Acceptance

Self-acceptance means knowing we are more than the unpleasant, frightening, and disturbing sensations that come into our mind. Many of us are quick to judge and criticize ourselves. We have heard in this group how strong this self-criticism can become, and how living with psychosis can lead people to feel different from others, or feel they have less value or are less human than others.

If we can learn to accept these experiences as part of being human, as just a part of who we are, we come to see we are more than the voices, images, thoughts, memories, feelings, and other sensations that come into our mind, that they do not define us, and that we have just as much value as other people. Self-acceptance involves letting go of judging ourselves for having these experiences, choosing to be kinder to ourselves, just as we would be to others.

Please make a note of one or two things you learned in Session 6:

____

____

____

____

____

____

____

Home Practice

As best you can:

- *Notice judging*—of your experiences and times when you are judging yourself
- *Notice acceptance*—of any moments when you can let these judgments go, accepting, in this moment, that this is my experience right now; notice how this feels

(continued)

From *Mindfulness for Psychosis: A Group Therapy Approach*, by Paul Chadwick, Katherine Newman-Taylor, and Nicola Abba. Copyright © 2027 The Guilford Press. Permission to photocopy this material, or to download and print enlarged versions (*www.guilford.com/chadwick-materials*), is granted to purchasers of this book for personal use or use with clients; see copyright page for details.

- *Practice guided mindfulness*—listen to the 10-minute audio recording, daily if possible
- *Notice moments of mindfulness*—"checking in with ourselves" (tuning into the sensations of breathing, anytime, anywhere), noticing moments of joy and connection (what are these for you?), and practicing ABC at difficult times (*awareness*—of what's happening right now, *breathing*—take a few natural breaths, *choice*—how do you want to respond right now in this moment?)

Week 6 Diary

Over the week, jot down anything you notice or learn from practicing mindfulness between sessions. You may wish to share your reflections with the group in the next session:

12

Sessions 7 and 8: Taking Mindful Steps toward Personal Recovery

The theme for the final two sessions conveys how group members' emerging sense of acceptance, of psychosis sensations, and of themselves further enables and motivates people to make changes in their day-to-day lives—changes that are already underway by this point in the program. This includes embedding mindfulness practice in ways that work for them and commencing (or recommencing) activities that give a sense of achievement, connection, and enjoyment. Over the final sessions, we encourage and validate ways in which people are reclaiming their lives and autonomy. While specific steps are determined by each person, facilitators draw out the common process of people freeing themselves from the grip of unpleasant psychosis sensations through increased hope, agency, and self-acceptance, and engaging in the lives they want to lead.

In these final sessions, we embrace a wider focus on mindfulness in daily life and discuss practical ways to sustain practice (which will reflect local context and opportunities; see Chapter 13). At the same time, it is important not to lose sight of the primary focus of the program—for people to learn to relate mindfully to psychosis sensations. Facilitators continue to guide and consolidate understanding of the impact of habitual reactivity and mindful responding.

Facilitating Group Factors in Sessions 7 and 8

The ending of even a relatively short-term group can elicit strong and contrasting feelings. Facilitators listen for and validate these feelings. Where this is likely to support group members' understanding of mindfulness, facilitators may also share some of their own feelings about the ending. We are also attending to the planned session structure, designed to continue to foster the unfolding process of change in mindfulness for psychosis groups.

Toward the end of the program, for many people the four group factors have become tightly interwoven as aspects of an overarching group process. Facilitators now reinforce group factors by highlighting examples from day-to-day life as much as from group sessions. In this way the group factors can become internalized processes no longer confined to the group setting.

Universality

As facilitators, we continue gently to reinforce universality that is both experience based (e.g., hearing voices and seeing images, moments of joy and connection), and person based (e.g., recognizing aspects of common humanity: "*We all* . . ."). Sharing feelings and concerns about the group ending, and noting acts of kindness and altruism, are further opportunities to strengthen universality (e.g., "*There was a lot of support from everybody to everybody today*"). Facilitators use open questions to prompt reflection with an increasing emphasis on person-based universality—for example: "*I remember at the start of the group how many of you felt different from other people, set apart from others. I wonder, how are you feeling now?*" People now start to affirm: "*I'm not different, I'm a person like everyone else*" and facilitators may share their pleasure in hearing these responses—for example: "*It's really good to hear that, Kamal.*"

During inquiry, we also look for opportunities to note that we all have times when we can be more accepting and times when we are more critical of ourselves; there is universality in recognizing that we are all prey to moments of self-judgment. Facilitators emphasize the benefit of greater balance in these moments of acceptance and judgment, in contrast to previous dominance of self-criticism, and support understanding that who we are (the self) is continually changing and evolving, never fixed.

Cohesion

As universality and hope continue to grow, so too does group cohesion. We foster this as people begin to reclaim their lives. For example:

> *"This group has really built my confidence. Hearing how everyone has started to make changes, and all the support from everyone here—it's made all the difference."*—USHA

Facilitators listen for and reflect on group members coming together to support one another, as well as learning for oneself. As above (for universality), acts of kindness and understanding that people show one another foster group cohesion, and we have observed altruism to be a powerful restorative experience, especially for people prone to paranoia and suspiciousness who have hitherto avoided others for fear of anticipated harm. Facilitators now encourage a gradual and targeted approach to establishing safety and cohesion in everyday life. For example:

> *"In earlier sessions, we heard how mistrusting everyone was isolating and keeping you locked into feelings of fear, paranoia, and confusion. We're now starting to hear how some of you are feeling safe enough to trust others and be yourselves a little more."*

In anticipation of ending the group, some may experience a transient increase in mistrust and feeling unsafe—that is, a return to the psychosis-driven feelings that dominated at the start of the group. We frame this as an understandable response to ending and uncertainty, and listen for examples of cohesion developed within the group generalizing to daily life. We encourage group members to trust their capacity to connect with and support other people in daily life.

Hope

For many, there is a growing sense of hope and empowerment that can be directed toward personal recovery and engagement in a valued life. Hope is expressed when people talk about "*not letting these voices stop me*," where earlier they described the same voices as omnipotent: "*ruling my life.*" At this stage in the program, some people are making important, often unanticipated changes in their day-to-day lives—for example:

> *"Twice I actually went to my local pub, where I used to go, and sat outside and had a pint in the sunshine. I haven't done that in ages; I was really delighted."*—GREG

Facilitators highlight that people's hope is moving beyond the possibility of coping better with psychosis, to broader expectations for personal recovery and living well even with psychosis experiences. We are careful not to suggest any need for what could be seen as *big* behavioral changes over these final sessions (or beyond): steps toward personal recovery are often *small* (in others' eyes) yet personally significant (e.g., going to the local pub) and facilitators encourage a continuation of this approach.

Being Myself More Fully

By this stage of the program, universality and being oneself more fully often become inseparable. Discovering that "*I am not different*" (universality) encourages people to continue expressing and being themselves in the group—perhaps sharing personal attributes, experiences, and hopes for the future. Having these contributions valued and accepted in the group further strengthens universality. The more of themselves that people bring to the group, the stronger becomes the metacognitive insight that "*I am more than the psychosis—I am more than these voices, images, thoughts, memories, and feelings—these are just a part of who I am.*"

In these final sessions, we ask about opportunities outside the group that are safe, supportive, and allow people to express and be themselves more fully day-to-day. Reflections in the opening check-in often provide examples of exactly this. We validate these while noting that for all of us, the degree to which we feel able to be ourselves varies with the setting, others present, and how we are feeling at that time. As with all the group factors, our ability to be ourselves more fully ebbs and flows. We encourage people to use informal mindfulness practices as an in-the-moment guide as they navigate being themselves more fully, noticing and accepting times when this does not feel possible, such as when this would leave them feeling too exposed and vulnerable.

SESSION GUIDANCE

Sessions 7 and 8 Structure

1. Opening the session
2. Review mindfulness practice over the week—habitual reactivity and mindful responding through formal practice and moments of mindfulness
3. First core mindfulness practice
4. Inquiry focused on first practice
5. *Session 7 psychoeducation:* the process of change in mindfulness for psychosis

   Session 8 psychoeducation: mindful steps toward recovery—the group ending and how to continue to practice

[Optional break]

6. Second core mindfulness practice
7. Inquiry focused on second practice and session learning points
8. Closing the session and home practice

Handouts

- Session handout

Opening the Session

We open each session by warmly welcoming group members, noting the session number and how many remain. We outline the session theme and structure as usual. For example:

> "*It's good to see you all. Today is our seventh/final session—our time together has gone quickly. As usual, we'll do two mindfulness practices with time for discussion. Today, we'll also go back over the process of learning mindfulness—stepping back and allowing difficult voices, images, thoughts, memories, and feelings to come into awareness; choosing not to react; and becoming more accepting of these experiences and ourselves. In the final session we'll share ideas about ways to support you to keep practicing mindfulness after the group has ended. First, let's start by hearing how you got on practicing mindfulness over the past week.*"

Check-In on Mindfulness Practice

At this stage in the program, most people are experiencing moments of each of the three main stages of the process of change in mindfulness for psychosis: *stepping back*, *choice*, and *acceptance* (see Chapter 3). There is a wide range of ways that people assimilate and practice mindfulness. Some use mindfulness as an ad hoc coping strategy when distressed by psychosis sensations and other stressors. Some develop a daily personal practice and draw on the attitudinal qualities of mindfulness to shape how they live their lives. As facilitators, we appreciate however group members choose to engage with mindfulness; our role is to introduce people to the practice, and support and trust them to make use of mindfulness in ways that work for them at this point in their life. It is important that facilitators keep this in mind at the check-in.

Group members have usually found ways to practice both formally and informally, and give examples of each. We ask about ways in which people are embedding mindfulness in their lives, the impact this is having on how people relate to psychosis sensations, and behavioral changes in people's daily life in line with personal hopes and goals for recovery. Initial changes often result in motivation and confidence to try further changes. For example:

> "*If I can go to the local pub, maybe I could try going to the local supermarket.*"—GREG

We are careful to appreciate all change equally, whether this is returning to paid employment or returning to the local pub. We emphasize that people are taking the steps that are important and right for them at this time. Prompting reflection on others' comments can be useful to help people recognize the progress they have made—for example: "*What was it like to hear others talking about what you'd achieved this week?*"

In terms of informal practice, at this stage we not only encourage people to be open to moments of joy and connection but actively seek out such opportunities—for example: "*When do you feel these moments of joy and connection in your lives? [Pause] How can you give yourself the best chance to experience these moments, day-to-day?*"

This will be different for each person. As an example, at the end of the program, Kamal still found being with other people stressful and triggered paranoia, but volunteering at an animal sanctuary had become a regular source of joy and connection. We listen carefully across sessions for the contexts in which each person experiences joy and connection, and highlight these.

As the group factors strengthen, people share a wide range of difficult and joyful experiences. We both encourage this and remain mindful of time! Supporting self-acceptance is a primary focus for the second half of the program, and we may link reflections during the check-in with self-acceptance—for example: *"Did anyone notice any moments over the past week of feeling more accepting of themselves? Moments of feeling OK with how you are doing or who you are?"*

Guiding the Core Mindfulness Practices

In the final two sessions, we weave in phrases that emphasize practicing together, and naming the three main elements of the core process of change. Prior to the first practice in each of the final sessions, we may take a moment to encourage people to commit fully to practicing together and supporting one another—for example: *"So, as we close our eyes, let's really give ourselves this time to practice together. Let's commit to practicing mindfulness together, to being as present as we can be for these few minutes."*

Additionally, we seek to name the three main elements of the core process of change to embed this understanding for group members. While we are sensitive to the unique nature of each group, we are careful to mention *stepping back*, *choice*, and *acceptance* during the guidance to align the core mindfulness practice, inquiry, and the process of change explicitly. For example:

> *"We are not trying to force our attention to stay on the breath. As best we can, we choose to be open to and accepting of whatever we experience, whether it is pleasant, unpleasant, or neutral. For these few minutes, if we can, allow each of these sensations to come fully into awareness, and then pass or fade into the background, without reacting to them. Then each time allowing our awareness gently to return and rest again in the sensations of breathing.*
>
> *"You may find that difficult voices, images, thoughts, feelings, and other sensations come back again a few moments later. Each time stepping back to allow the sensations to come fully into awareness and then*

pass or fade, choosing to let these come and go without reacting, and as best you can, accepting the sensations and yourself in this moment.

"Often, we find we have been lost, maybe struggling with voices, caught up in rumination or worry. We all get lost like this. There is no need to judge yourself. When this happens, as best we can, we notice how it feels in the body, how it feels emotionally, to let go of this struggle and reconnect with the sensations of breathing. Stepping back and choosing to accept that in this moment, this is my experience. Just resting our awareness in the sensations of the breath as we breathe in and as we breathe out."

Facilitators will make minor adaptations to the core mindfulness script to emphasize key points relevant to the stage of the program, and group members' development of mindful responses to psychosis sensations. These final sessions offer valuable opportunities to deepen people's mindfulness practice.

Facilitating the Two Periods of Inquiry

In Sessions 7 and 8, we focus on consolidating learning and extending application of mindfulness to day-to-day life and personal recovery, rather than introducing new ideas. Facilitators seek to recognize and build progress within and outside the group. One way of consolidating learning is to draw out the three main elements of the process of change in mindfulness for psychosis (as well as naming these in the guided mindfulness practice, as outlined above): *stepping back*, *choosing how to respond*, and *accepting unpleasant psychosis sensations and ourselves*. Particular attention often needs to be paid to acceptance, building on Sessions 5 and 6.

In terms of applying mindfulness to day-to-day life and steps toward personal recovery, the balance of inquiry often shifts from reflections on practice in sessions to (1) examples of mindful responding and acceptance in daily life and (2) behavioral changes these often initiate (rather than detailed mapping of what happened during practice).

In these final sessions, we continue to frame reflective discussion, bringing attention to key moments of habitual reactivity and mindful responding, and guiding discovery. This often involves asking for others' views—we are comfortable acknowledging when we are struggling to put a point into words and asking for the group's help with this—for example: *"That's an interesting question, what do others think about how to bring mindfulness into day-to-day life?"*

In Session 7, facilitators close the second period of inquiry in the usual way, inviting people to share something they have learned or that stands out for them from the session, and, if time permits, offering a brief reflection on the theme of acceptance. In the final session, the invitation is to share what stands out from the program as a whole (and this is prompted in the final handout). Facilitators usually wait to the end of the session to give a brief reflection of their own when closing the session.

Focusing on Moments of Mindfulness Practice That Support Learning

In Sessions 7 and 8, the focus on moments of mindfulness and learning from this widens to incorporate more examples from day-to-day life—whether through formal or informal mindfulness practice, or through the behavior changes we increasingly see toward the end of the group—as well as practices within these final sessions. We note how repeated moments of choosing to respond mindfully in daily life further strengthen people's sense of agency, self-acceptance, and personal recovery.

Attitude toward Practice

As some group members become concerned about the end of the group, it is essential that facilitators continue to embody the attitudinal qualities that support the group factors and process of change—authenticity, acceptance, and trust—as best they can. As a reminder, it is helpful to tune into these in the minutes before each of the final two sessions, acknowledging that the ending of the group may bring up questions and concerns for facilitators too (which should be brought to supervision). We do not need to finish brilliantly! We do not need to rehearse all that has gone before. We follow the session structure and do our best to focus discussion on key points that arise, accepting that some material from previous sessions will not be covered; we trust group members to continue to utilize what they have learned from the group in ways that work for them. As best we can, we relax into being fully present and ourselves for these final sessions.

In terms of shaping attitude to practice for group members, we continue to model and encourage a gentle and accepting approach to mindfulness practice. We listen for opportunities to highlight that while our ability to respond mindfully inevitably ebbs and flows, we can recover from setbacks by starting again and again. Additionally, some have started to notice that difficult days and spells of reactivity become fewer, briefer, and less intense, as they build mindfulness practice into a daily routine, and know in moments when psychosis and other unpleasant sensations intrude into awareness, that "*This will pass.*"

In these last sessions, we gently reinforce the importance of sustained and steady practice. This is particularly important toward the end of the group, to encourage people to build mindfulness practice into their daily lives. Some people may find that psychosis sensations have become less frequent and preoccupying, leading to a belief that mindfulness practice may no longer be necessary. Where appropriate, we emphasize the link between mindfulness and any easing of psychosis sensations, as well as the value of ongoing practice to strengthen readiness for any future setbacks and challenges in life. Regular practice is also for many of us a rare time to give our mind and body some rest.

Guiding Discovery Related to Habitual Distressing Reactions and Mindful Responding

In Sessions 7 and 8, we seek to guide discovery linked to material covered in all sessions. We ask the group open, broad questions to reinforce key metacognitive insights about psychosis, habitual reactivity, mindful responding, and the self. Pulling together previous material in this way (rather than listing key points) enables people to articulate and thereby strengthen learning in ways that work for them:

- *"What have you learned about unpleasant voices, images, thoughts, and feelings from being in the group?"*
- *"What does being mindful mean for you?"*
- *"What is the impact of trying to avoid unpleasant sensations?"*
- *"How does it feel when you get lost in reacting? How does it feel in moments of mindfulness—when you can step back, choose not to react, and be more accepting?"*
- *"How do you feel when you tune into moments of mindfulness in daily life?"*
- *"What is the impact of constantly being self-critical and judgmental?"*
- *"How does being mindful help?"*
- *"What have you learned about yourselves from being in the group and practicing mindfulness together?"*

Drawing Attention to Unhelpful Metacognitive Beliefs and Helpful Metacognitive Insights

Prior to the final sessions, it can be helpful for facilitators to remind themselves of common metacognitive beliefs that maintain distressing reactions, and metacognitive insights that support mindful responding (see Chapter 2, Table 2.1). People will of course describe these in slightly different ways given their experience and what fits for them.

People often reflect on how psychosis and other unpleasant sensations, when stripped of distressing reactivity, *deflate*—lose much of their perceived power and no longer dominate their lives as before. Many people are less distressed and frightened by psychosis sensations, which now draw their attention and preoccupy them less. Sandra described how previously, when traveling on the subway, her voices were "*there all the time*" and that she would be lost "*in another world*" and miss her stop. Having learned to practice mindfulness regularly, she described how "*The voices are still there but I know where I am, I see the people around me, I get off when I need to.*" Sandra found that she could choose to let go of the struggle and feel calmer, stronger, more in control.

Psychosis sensations may persist and remain unpleasant. However, many people come to recognize that while others have not lived with intrusions and disturbance of the magnitude and devastation experienced by people with psychosis, everyone has unpleasant intrusions, and the metacognitive belief that "*I am fundamentally the same as other people.*"

When people reflect on change over the course of the group, we seek to frame habitual reactivity as inevitable and necessary ways of coping in the past—as universal instinctive reactions to unpleasant, frightening, and disturbing events. We acknowledge once more how voices, images, thoughts, memories, and other sensations are often a result of earlier aversive or traumatic events, and encourage *an accepting, compassionate attitude toward our habitual reactivity*, both in the past and when these reemerge at times of stress.

While we listen for and reinforce individualized versions of metacognitive insights that support mindful responding, facilitators remind the group that there is no aim to be entirely free of avoidance, struggle, and judgment—we seek choice and balance. Mindfulness supports us to learn to recognize habitual cycles of reactivity, to step back and choose to respond differently, and how each feels in the body and mind, and emotionally.

Moments of Mindful Responding

We attend to examples of habitual cycles of reactivity and mindful responding, both in group practices and day-to-day life, drawing out how each feels in the body and mind, and emotionally. We gently contrast these to draw out key metacognitive insights—for example: "*What difference does it make to step back and respond mindfully, to accept these unpleasant images and sense of confusion?*"

We draw attention to moments of joy and connection linked to mindful responding, elicit how these feel, and what people learn about themselves from these moments. This also reinforces the message that we can be mindful of all experiences, not just stressful, unpleasant ones—for example: "*How do you feel in these moments of connection, and what does this say about you?*"

We continue to attend to moments of decentered awareness of the sensations of breathing, perhaps when unpleasant voices, images, thoughts, and other sensations move to the background—for example: "*How does it feel to spend a few moments of resting awareness in the sensations of breathing?*"

People often note the restorative quality of time spent resting our mind and body, and describe versions of the metacognitive insights that "*Not reacting is possible and can feel calming and peaceful*" and "*When I'm grounded in my breath, I can bear the psychosis.*"

Balance, Evolving Self-Acceptance, and Personal Recovery

During inquiry in the final sessions, it can be helpful to talk in terms of developing balance. This applies to mindfulness practice—finding ways to practice that work for us and can be sustained over the long term, and to habitual reactivity and mindful responding—knowing that we will have setbacks at times of stress or when we let regular practice slip, but can always begin again and again.

In terms of the ebb and flow of judgment and self-acceptance, we look for opportunities to highlight how we all have moments of self-criticism and moments of self-acceptance. What mindfulness offers is a more balanced sense of self (Chadwick, 2006). Greater acceptance comes when group members start to let go of defining themselves in relation to malevolent voices, perceived persecutors, and so on, to recognize a universality with others, and to actively reengage with all that gives them a sense of achievement, connection, and enjoyment.

In these last two sessions, group members often talk about the importance of group factors in supporting self-acceptance, as much as formal and informal mindfulness practice. Through hearing how others have lived with and been affected by psychosis, and having experienced the support that others willingly offer, many group members develop a more balanced, and fuller (more nuanced) sense of self, understanding that change is inevitable and growth is always possible. This contrasts with the profound sense of dehumanization that dominates many people with psychosis. Group members are starting to experience what it means to be a person like others, and understand that there is room for psychosis sensations to be part of who they are, whether these persist or pass—for example: "*When I accept my psychosis and myself, I feel more human.*"

With greater balance and evolving self-acceptance, people start to make the changes they would like to see in their lives. We encourage people to use moments of self-acceptance as signposts when taking steps toward personal recovery. If this does not come up in the inquiry, we can prompt discussion, perhaps by asking the group "*In those moments when you feel more accepting of yourselves, are there things you feel you would like to do more of in your life, things that feel right and important to you?*"

Common Challenges to Practice at Sessions 7 and 8

At this point, most people are encountering few if any new challenges to practicing mindfulness during sessions, though challenges faced in earlier sessions often resurface, particularly regarding acceptance of psychosis and the self (see previous challenges tables as a reminder). Occasionally people think they no longer need to practice because things are going well, and psychosis sensations have become less frequent and distressing. While being careful not to be alarmist, we gently reinforce the link with regular practice over the course of the program, and the value of ongoing practice to ensure readiness for any setbacks and difficult days ahead. We might comment on how we also find having a regular practice helps us cope better at times of stress. The major challenge raised in the final sessions concerns people's ability to continue to practice mindfulness without the group. The major challenge raised in the final sessions concerns people's ability to continue to practice mindfulness without the group (see the following table).

Common Challenges Arising in Sessions 7 and 8, and Possible Responses

Challenges	Examples	Unhelpful metacognitive beliefs and judgments	Possible responses from facilitators
Concerns about practicing after the group has ended	*"I won't be able to practice mindfulness on my own, without the support of the people in the group."*	*"I'm too weak, don't have the strength others have."*	Validate—listen to and validate the range of feelings and concerns about the group ending.
		"There's something lacking in me."	Build universality and contextualize. *"It's understandable to have doubts and fears, perhaps some sadness, as we come to the end of the group, when this has been helpful, and you've connected with people here—I'm sure we all understand this."*
	"I won't be able to talk to people outside like I can talk to the people in the group—I'll be lonely and isolated again."	*"I don't have the support I'd need to keep going with mindfulness."*	Instill hope. *"For many people, once they've been able to say how they feel about the group ending, and hear others have similar concerns, they start to feel more hopeful about building on what they started here."* *"It's understandable to have worries and doubts about the ending. I wonder, are there any things that make you feel hopeful about the future? Anything you've learned here that you can build on?"* *"For many, these doubts pass, and they continue to practice mindfulness and to become kinder, more accepting of themselves."* *"If you do find you could use more support, as we discussed earlier, there are sources of support available."*
			Reinforce self-acceptance and agency. *"As we've talked about before, it's easy for us to think that there's something wrong or lacking with us and to doubt ourselves. But think about all you've done in just these last weeks, and what you are discovering about yourself."* *"I wonder, are there other ways to build connections with people outside the group and perhaps even practice with them?"*

In response, we discuss practical local options that we know and would recommend for ongoing support to practice mindfulness, such as Recovery College courses or aligned mindfulness groups hosted by known mental health charities (see Chapter 13 for decision making about what to recommend). We take care not to minimize the impact of the group ending for anyone finding this difficult.

Psychoeducation in Sessions 7 and 8

Psychoeducation in Sessions 7 and 8 is focused firmly on recognizing progress within and outside the group, consolidating learning, and anticipating next steps for personal recovery. As always, we take a conversational approach to outlining key points briefly, using examples from the group and inviting reflective discussion.

Session 7 psychoeducation outlines the process of change in mindfulness for psychosis (see Chapter 3) as a way to draw together all that has been covered in the group, recognize progress, and consolidate learning. For example:

> *"Today we'd like to look back over the last few weeks, and recap what we've covered. Over these sessions we've talked about how reacting to unpleasant, frightening, and disturbing sensations that come into our mind—with avoidance, rumination, worry, confrontation, and judgment—creates distress and is disempowering. These understandable reactions are making things worse, not better.*
>
> *"Stepping back and choosing to let unpleasant voices, images, thoughts, memories, and feelings come into awareness and then pass or fade, without reacting to them, leaves you feeling calmer, stronger, more in control. The more you are able and willing to accept these unpleasant sensations as just a part of your experience, and the more you accept yourselves, the less power and control the voices, images, thoughts, and so on have over you and your life.*
>
> *"Being in a group with other people who have similar experiences has helped you learn mindfulness and see that you are not different from other people. None of us can be mindful all the time; we all get caught up in reacting sometimes—maybe when thoughts or voices are stronger, or when we are tired or feeling unwell. It is important that we are kind to*

ourselves at these times, just as we would be to others who are struggling, and keep in mind that we all are doing the best we can.

"Does this make sense? It would be great to hear what you think about this."

Session 8 psychoeducation then focuses on ways to continue to practice, and how mindfulness can help day-to-day and support steps toward personal recovery. For example:

"Last session we talked about how being in this group has helped you learn mindfulness, and how seeing how much we all have in common has helped you be more accepting of your experiences and yourselves.

"Over the weeks we've seen how much each of you has been able to take what you've been learning here and apply this outside the group in your daily lives. You've been practicing mindfulness in many ways: listening to the recording, checking in with yourselves, noticing moments of joy, stepping back and not reacting when stressed, and becoming more accepting of yourselves. You've been finding how to fit mindfulness into your daily routine.

"We've seen how mindfulness and the group has supported you to reclaim your lives in ways that really matter to each of you [give examples]. When we are mindful and more accepting of ourselves, we often start to notice and recognize what we want to do more of in our lives and feel more able to take steps in line with our hopes and goals [give examples].

"Our hope in running this group is that this will help you be more accepting of yourselves, and feel empowered to take the steps that are important to you—to do the things that give you a sense of achievement, connection, and enjoyment. Now let's think together about how to keep this going after the group has finished."

Maintaining practice is important and we encourage group members to share strategies that have enabled them to embed mindfulness practice in their lives. The Session 7 handout prompts people to note any ideas, so we can suggest they look over these, share any that others may find helpful, and jot down any others that might work for them. We also emphasize the importance of keeping key learning from the group in mind, ask people how they have or might do this, and access this even at difficult times. People often share great ideas, such as using phones, journals (also highlighted in the final handout), notes on the refrigerator, or on a bedroom door, objects that represent self-acceptance or moments of joy—and some we have not encountered before.

Closing the Session, Home Practice, and Handouts

In Sessions 7 and 8, we encourage people to continue using the core mindfulness practice regularly—daily for those who have established a daily practice, and at least once each week. We also recommend ongoing ad hoc use of the three informal practices to maintain stepping back, choice, and acceptance in daily life. There is no need to make a last *big push* for more home practice—by now, group members know that we recommend regular sustained practice, and pushing for more may undermine this. We communicate our trust that each person is bringing mindfulness into their daily life in a way that works for them. For example:

> *"We've been impressed by how each of you have worked out how to bring mindfulness into your daily life, in ways that work for you. We encourage you to continue this, and keep looking for new ways, perhaps asking yourself: How could I be a little more mindful this week?"*

Distributing and describing the session handout is an opportunity to outline how some people like to keep a mindfulness journal to note their practice and any reflections. We also encourage people to review the previous handouts from time to time as a recap of the group, remind themselves of what they have learned, and extend the benefits of learning mindfulness for psychosis.

Finally, we offer a few closing words of our own. This is an authentic expression of our gratitude for the opportunity to get to know each person, to have been able to introduce them to mindfulness, and see how well they have made use of this. We say that we hope they will continue to use mindfulness in the ways that work for them.

Mindfulness Group: Session 7 Handout

Reacting to Psychosis Causes Distress

Today we reminded ourselves of the main points from the sessions so far: (1) how automatic it can be to react to unpleasant voices, images, thoughts, memories, feelings, and other sensations, with avoidance, struggle, and judgment; and (2) how reacting in these ways does not work well, creates distress, and feels disempowering. We can't control what comes into our mind, but by practicing mindfulness we can choose how we respond.

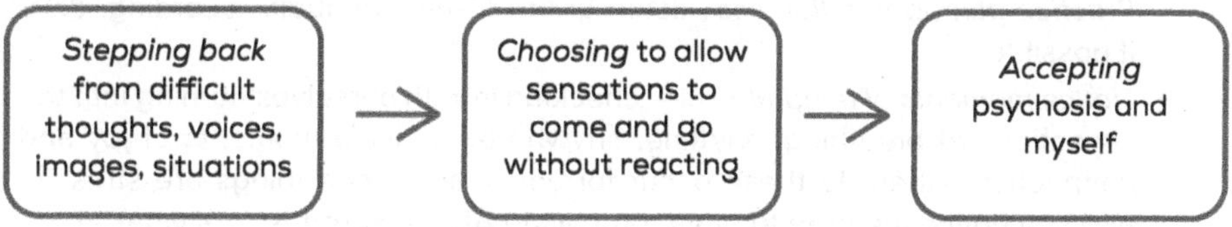

The Process of Change in Mindfulness for Psychosis

Stepping back and allowing unpleasant psychosis sensations to come into awareness while gently focusing on the sensations of the breath is the first step to mindful responding.

Choosing to allow sensations to come fully into awareness and then pass or fade without avoiding, struggling, or judging brings a sense of calm and peace.

Accepting these sensations as a part of your experience gives you more control of your mind and personal recovery. Accepting yourself eases suffering—learning that you are not different and much more than the psychosis.

Please make a note of one or two things you learned in Session 7:

(continued)

From *Mindfulness for Psychosis: A Group Therapy Approach*, by Paul Chadwick, Katherine Newman-Taylor, and Nicola Abba. Copyright © 2027 The Guilford Press. Permission to photocopy this material, or to download and print enlarged versions (*www.guilford.com/chadwick-materials*), is granted to purchasers of this book for personal use or use with clients; see copyright page for details.

Home Practice

This week, as best you can:

- *Notice judging*—of your experiences and yourself for having these experiences
- *Notice acceptance*—moments when you let these judgments go and accept the psychosis sensations and yourself; how does this feel?
- *Practice guided mindfulness*—listen to the 10-minute audio recording, daily if possible
- *Notice moments of mindfulness*—"checking in with ourselves" (tuning into the sensations of breathing, anytime, anywhere), noticing moments of joy and connection (when do these occur for you?), and when things are stressful and you notice the urge to react, practicing ABC (*awareness*—of what's happening right now, *breathing*—take a few natural breaths, *choice*—how do you want to respond right now in this moment?)

None of us is mindful all the time. There will be times when you get caught up in cycles of avoidance, worry, struggle, and judgment—maybe when the voices, images, thoughts, memories, or feelings are strong, or life becomes stressful. At these times, as best you can, show yourself the kindness and compassion you show others, reminding yourself that you are more than the psychosis.

Week 7 Diary

Over the week, jot down how you plan to continue to practice mindfulness once the group has ended:

____

____

____

____

____

____

____

____

Mindfulness Group: Session 8 Handout

Learning Mindfulness

It's hard to choose what to say in this final handout! Do reread the earlier handouts from time to time, to remind yourself of all we've covered. As the group comes to an end, we want to recognize how much you have supported one another to practice mindfulness and learn to be more accepting of psychosis and other unpleasant sensations, and of yourselves.

We've seen over the last weeks how each one of you has taken what you've learned in the group and applied this in your own lives—listening to the recording, checking in with yourselves during the day, enjoying moments of joy and connection, or stepping back and not reacting to difficult situations. You have brought mindfulness into your daily lives in ways that work for you.

Responding Mindfully

Learning to respond mindfully to psychosis takes effort and practice. Stepping back and choosing to accept that unpleasant sensations come to mind, letting these arise and then pass or fade, is empowering and gives you more control. There will be ups and downs, good days and difficult days. Mindfulness helps us recognize, with acceptance and kindness to ourselves, that we are doing our best to navigate our way through this.

Mindful Steps to Recovery

When feeling more empowered and accepting of ourselves, it is possible to take steps toward personal recovery—doing more of the things that really matter, that give you a sense of achievement, connection, or enjoyment that you may have stopped when struggling with psychosis. In this group, we've seen many examples of people reclaiming their lives in this way.

Our hope is that you will continue to practice mindfulness and that this gives you more choice, acceptance, and kindness in your lives, enabling each of you to live well with psychosis.

(continued)

From *Mindfulness for Psychosis: A Group Therapy Approach*, by Paul Chadwick, Katherine Newman-Taylor, and Nicola Abba. Copyright © 2027 The Guilford Press. Permission to photocopy this material, or to download and print enlarged versions (*www.guilford.com/chadwick-materials*), is granted to purchasers of this book for personal use or use with clients; see copyright page for details.

What Has Stood Out for You?

Looking back over all our group meetings, what stands out for you? What have you learned about the unpleasant voices, images, thoughts, memories, feelings, and other sensations that arise? What have you learned about yourself? Please write down whatever comes to mind:

____

____

____

____

____

____

Building a Regular Mindfulness Practice

As the group comes to an end, we invite you to commit to practicing mindfulness regularly, in ways that work for you. This might include listening to the 10-minute audio recording at least once or twice a week.

Moments of mindfulness; remember the practices to use in your daily life:

- *"Checking in with ourselves"*—tuning into the sensations of breathing, anytime, anywhere
- *Noticing moments of joy and connection*—really appreciating these when they arise
- *Practicing ABC when things are stressful and you feel you may react—awareness* of what's happening right now, taking a few natural *breaths*, and *choosing* how you want to respond in this moment

Mindfulness Journal

Many people find it helps to keep a mindfulness journal after the group has finished. In the journal you can make a brief note when you have practiced, jot down any reflections, or write down any important ways that mindfulness has been helpful to you day-to-day.

It has been a pleasure to meet and get to know each of you, and we hope mindfulness continues to be helpful to you in the future.

IV

Supporting Ongoing Recovery and Developing as Facilitators

13

Ongoing Support Beyond the Mindfulness for Psychosis Program

Toward the end of the program, facilitators are often asked if there is anything they can either offer themselves or recommend to support people to practice mindfulness after the program has finished. People usually ask this not because they have struggled to grasp mindfulness and want to try again but because something has changed and they are starting to see new possibilities.

When writing this book, we revisited the question of support beyond the eight-session program. We believe strongly that if people wish to continue to develop a mindful relationship with psychosis in their daily life, then some form of ongoing support is likely to be helpful. In this chapter we discuss different options that we recommend as ways to sustain and deepen understanding and practice of mindfulness after the 8-week program. All options that we recommend align with the principles of mindfulness for psychosis articulated in this book and are ones that people have reported finding useful.

Group Members' Concern about the Program Ending: What Comes Next?

As a group approaches the final sessions, people often experience a range of emotions. Usually there is a measure of hope, gratitude to the group, and emerging trust in mindfulness, alongside feelings about the group coming to an end, and some apprehension and concern about continuing without the support of the group.

Concerns include general feelings of loss and apprehension that commonly arise when any cohesive group therapy comes to an end. People also express concerns about how to sustain and deepen their mindfulness practice, both formally and informally, who they'll be able to talk to about these experiences, and how to manage the risk of sliding back into the grip of distressing reactivity to psychosis sensations (the left side of the two-circles model; see Chapter 2, Figure 2.1). People may feel concerned about losing the combination of guided mindfulness practices, reflective group discussions, and being part of a group that has supported steps toward personal recovery. They may also worry about losing the gains made toward accepting both their psychosis and themselves, and reclaiming the lives they want to lead. Individuals' personal practice and development of mindful responses to psychosis (the right side of the two-circles model) can feel precarious at this point, as can benefits to their well-being and wider lives. Group members are often worried about becoming isolated again, losing connection with other people and moments of joy in their lives.

All these feelings and concerns can be explored in the group. Time is spent throughout the program, and particularly in Sessions 7 and 8, thinking about how to embed mindfulness in daily life. It is also helpful for facilitators to have considered (1) people's likely individual needs toward the end of the eight-session program, and (2) local options available, to be ready to offer recommendations for ongoing support if requested.

Guiding Principles When Recommending Options for Ongoing Support

As clinicians, we do all we can to minimize risk of potential harms when delivering any psychological intervention. When making recommendations for ways to support ongoing practice after the program has ended, the same professional responsibility regarding safety applies.

The 8-week mindfulness for psychosis program is based on a clear theoretical framework of mindful responding to psychosis (see Chapter 2) and how to progress toward this (see Chapter 3). Sessions incorporate brief (10-minute) guided practices designed for people with current distressing psychosis that include frequent (grounding) comments from facilitators—this is the foundational practice in all sessions. Sessions are run as therapy groups rather than large-scale skills classes; more time is devoted to reflective group discussion than to formal mindfulness practice, and facilitators attend to key group processes (universality, cohesion and belonging, hope, and being oneself more fully) as well as the session content. Regarding home practice, we emphasize choice and accept however much or little practice people manage each week. These features are intended to ensure that mindfulness practice occurs within an accepting and validating interpersonal group context, and to minimize any possible risk or harm.

We only recommend options that align with the need to (1) understand the distinction between habitual reactivity and mindful responding to psychosis; (2) incorporate brief mindfulness practices and inquiry; (3) emphasize choice and acceptance, and allow people to learn at their own pace; and (4) support universality and other key group factors. It is important that facilitators check that any options align with these points before making any recommendations.

Option 1: Gain Further Experience of Group-Based Mindfulness Therapy or Training

One popular option is for people to gain further experience of group-based mindfulness practice either by repeating the eight-session program, or by attending a mindfulness course or drop-in group that is *well aligned with the theory and principles of the program.* Mindfulness for psychosis facilitators may themselves also be involved in other local provision such as Recovery College and Recovery Education Center mindfulness groups and health care mindfulness groups, easing the transition from the 8-week program.

Repeating the Eight-Session Program

In many mindfulness for psychosis groups, we have had a small number of people returning for the second or even third time. Some return with little or no break between groups, gaining fairly continuous engagement, whereas others join a subsequent group after a break of several weeks or months. Most people who chose to repeat the program have engaged well and benefited the first time. People usually repeat the program to deepen their learning and practice, strengthen a growing ability to respond mindfully to psychosis and day-to-day stressors, and strengthen an emerging sense of self-acceptance, agency, and connection in daily life.

We raise the possibility of repeating the program as just one of a number of options that some people have found helpful. If a group includes someone who is repeating the program, then this possibility is evident from the outset, and often this person will have commented on the value of returning for them. We are careful not to suggest that repeating the program is expected or necessary, or the right or best thing to do. For many, attending one 8-week program is sufficient (at least for the time being). If an individual has missed several sessions and we think they would benefit (and could attend more consistently), we might suggest this directly.

People who repeat the 8-week program bring valuable experience and learning that can benefit other group members and facilitators. People who attend for a second or third time have much to contribute about the process of learning to relate mindfully to psychosis, including how to face challenges and bumps in the road. Additionally, having a person in the group who clearly values the opportunity to continue practicing mindfulness, and may be further along in their personal recovery, can be a source of hope and motivation for others. Facilitators also benefit—people with prior experience of the eight-session program often reinforce key points and learning through powerful personal experience and help establish a group culture of hope and the possibility of change.

Attending a Local Recovery College Mindfulness Course

Mindfulness courses offered through Recovery Colleges, or Recovery Education Centres, can be an excellent next step for people who have completed the eight-session program. The ethos of these colleges—adopting an educational approach to learning to live well with mental health conditions—aligns with the philosophy and practice of mindfulness for psychosis groups. Recovery Colleges are usually able to support and accommodate people with distressing voices, images, paranoia, and other psychosis experiences. While mindfulness courses vary across these colleges, all are likely to be comparatively short and include brief mindfulness practices and reflective group discussion. We encourage facilitators to attend a local Recovery College mindfulness course to gauge suitability for people with psychosis who have attended the 8-week program. In our experience, these colleges also welcome guidance and support to ensure courses offered are accessible and beneficial to people with psychosis.

A further strength of Recovery Colleges as a source of postgroup support is the centrality of co-production and co-facilitation between professionals and people living with mental ill health. Two of us have had the opportunity to co-facilitate Recovery College courses alongside people who combine lived experience of psychosis and trauma with training expertise, and have seen time and again how valuable their presence and guidance can be in engendering hope for participants' own personal recovery. If you are running a mindfulness for psychosis group, you might also consider contributing to a co-delivered Recovery College course that could support people beyond this.

In addition to being a source of ongoing support following the eight-session program, Recovery College mindfulness courses can be a pathway *to* the program. Fostering good working relationships with local Recovery Colleges and becoming familiar with the courses available can also help facilitators support people with psychosis navigate the range of options available in their area.

Attending an Ongoing Drop-In Mindfulness Group

Where available and suitable, an ongoing drop-in mindfulness group can be another excellent option for people to consolidate gains from the eight-session program. We developed mindfulness for psychosis groups within busy, overstretched National Health Service (NHS) mental health services in the United Kingdom. Offering any ongoing postgroup support is always a resource challenge. An open drop-in mindfulness group can work well.

Our experience of running a drop-in mindfulness group was as one of a number of activities run in a community mental health day center facility. We worked with the center to set up the drop-in sessions partly to support people's ongoing practice following the eight-session program. All sessions were open to any service user, family member, or carer attending the center. People attended when this suited them, signed in at reception, and joined any of the activities that were running. Time-intensive administration was therefore not needed from the facilitator. Meeting regularly for an hour each week provided a predictable and effective source of ongoing support for many people who had completed the eight-session mindfulness for psychosis program. Locating the group in a community mental health facility meant there were always trained clinical staff present who held overall responsibility for wider governance and risk issues. The drop-in group ran for several years, and being open to all gave opportunities to extend universality beyond people with psychosis.

The format used in the eight-session program also provides a useful basis for structuring open drop-in sessions: (1) a brief check-in on any mindfulness practice over the week; (2) a 10-minute core mindfulness practice; (3) inquiry, sometimes incorporating brief psychoeducation; (4) a briefer second practice; and (5) encouragement to explore formal and informal practices in everyday life.

Benefits of Attending Further Group-Based Mindfulness Therapy or Training

Repeating the eight-session program, attending a Recovery College mindfulness course, or joining ongoing drop-in sessions can strengthen people's sense of connection with others and bring collective benefits, as well as building individuals' ability to respond mindfully to psychosis and in wider daily life.

Throughout this book we have stressed the importance of two fundamentally humanizing therapeutic processes at the heart of mindfulness for psychosis groups: *universality* (discovering others have similar difficulties) and *connection* (with everyday moments of joy, and with other people). Attending further group-based mindfulness options (as outlined above) provides people with distressing psychosis additional opportunities to see that others share their experiences and struggles, and to connect with other people.

Repeating the 8-week program gives further opportunities for recognizing commonality of experience and connecting with a new group of people with psychosis. Recovery College courses typically attract people with a range of mental health conditions, not just psychosis, and may also be open to local health care staff and the public, offering even broader opportunity for universality and connection. This is particularly important given the stigma associated with mental ill health, and psychosis specifically, which people with psychosis internalize just as much as others in society. Similarly, community drop-in mindfulness groups are likely to be transdiagnostic and provide rich opportunities to deepen a sense of universality and connection, irrespective of diagnosis.

Option 2: Access an Aligned Psychological Therapy for Psychosis

There are many psychological therapies that benefit people with psychosis: those with an established evidence base and others based on an emerging body of literature. Here we consider therapies that incorporate principles of mindfulness and acceptance, and are well placed to consolidate and extend gains from mindfulness for psychosis groups.

Psychological therapies that are well aligned with the eight-session program include cognitive-behavioral therapy (CBT), acceptance and commitment therapy (ACT), and person-based cognitive therapy (PBCT). Increasingly, clinicians weave in mindfulness principles and practice into CBT where indicated by the person's individualized formulation—for example, where rumination keeps people stuck in cycles of unhelpful appraisals and reactions to voices or paranoia (Newman-Taylor & Abba, 2013, 2015, 2018). ACT incorporates mindfulness (and other *defusion*) exercises to enable people to step back from patterns of reactivity and choose alternative responses in line with their values and goals (Hayes, 2002; O'Donoghue et al., 2018). PBCT uses the same core mindfulness practice as the eight-session mindfulness for psychosis program (Chadwick, 2006).

Each of these approaches, and potentially others, emphasizes self-acceptance and acceptance of current psychosis to forge a meaningful and socially connected life, and support people to live well with psychosis. Not only are these psychological therapies suitable ways to build on gains from the 8-week program, the 8-week program can be excellent preparation for individual therapies including CBT, ACT, and PBCT by providing a foundation in mindfulness and self-acceptance grounded in universality.

Option 3: Practice with a Partner, Family Member, or Professional

From time to time, people attending the group get in the habit of practicing guided mindfulness outside the group with a partner, family member, friend, or mental health professional (e.g., a key worker). Using the core practice in this way has generally worked well, embedding mindfulness practice in the person's daily routine, and providing additional motivation and support through having someone else in their lives practicing alongside them. It can also be empowering for the person with psychosis sometimes to guide and support the other person learning mindfulness.

Practicing with a partner, family member, friend, or professional can also be combined with gaining further experience of group-based mindfulness therapy or training through Recovery College courses or drop-in sessions, where these are available and open to others as well as people with psychosis. Attending these together can strengthen and sustain ongoing joint practice at home.

Coda

We believe the form and context of mindfulness *as adapted for people with psychosis* in this program to be consistent with and reflect the intention of its Buddhist origins, and not in any way be *denatured*. Nonetheless, we do not recommend that people deepen their understanding and practice of mindfulness gained from the 8-week program with traditional meditation practices, or by attending meditation retreats or meditation centers. These traditions commonly include prolonged periods of practice, silence, or isolation, which may bring associated risks of harm for people with psychosis.

Historically, a small number of case reports have highlighted harmful effects of traditional meditation practices for people with psychosis. These harmful effects were largely related to people with (or vulnerable to) psychosis spending periods of time engaged in extended and traditional forms of meditation practice with limited social interaction or guidance. The mindfulness for psychosis program presented in this book has been designed not only to maximize potential therapeutic benefits but to address possible risks associated with lengthy practices, too little guidance, and social or sensory isolation.

Mindfulness for psychosis groups were developed and evaluated within secular health care settings. We do not draw on the language of Buddhist ethics, religion, psychology, or ontology. The structure and process of the 8-week program embeds the understanding and practice of mindfulness within a conceptual framework that incorporates a psychological understanding of psychosis, therapeutic group processes, and how people learn to free themselves from the tyranny of psychosis.

The options we have recommended are included because they are well aligned with the context, structure, and process of the 8-week program, and because people with psychosis have reported finding them to be beneficial to build on gains from the mindfulness for psychosis group. There will of course be other suitable options that we have not included. Additionally, if people are looking for different forms of support, there are other avenues to explore, such as peer support (e.g., Proctor et al., 2019), which also fosters acceptance, hope, and universality. Finally, we have not recommended any specific online resources, but do give all who attend the program free recordings of the core mindfulness practice (facilitators can use either their own recording of the "Core mindfulness practice," or the version we provide in Track 1 at *www.guilford.com/chadwick-materials*; see Appendix 9.1), and encourage ongoing practice. Session handouts can also be reviewed and rehearsed, independently or with others, such as clinicians or family, for ongoing support and guidance.

14

Preparation and Development as Group Facilitators

This chapter addresses the important question of what professional training and experience are considered a prerequisite to facilitating mindfulness for psychosis groups. We also offer guidance and resources to support ongoing learning and development for facilitators. Our intentions are to (1) benefit people with psychosis by ensuring that mindfulness is offered in a way that is safe and consistent with the underlying theory, and therefore therapeutic; and (2) support facilitators' own well-being and professional development.

We expect that anyone planning to offer the eight-session program has read this book and is able to adhere to the guidance and group manual. This includes being able to share the central frameworks and guide in-session practices. For newer facilitators, we strongly recommend working with a co-facilitator—ideally someone with prior experience of these groups. At least one of you should have therapeutic experience working with people with psychosis.

These recommendations pertain to facilitating mindfulness for psychosis groups as described in this book, following the eight-session manual in line with the underlying theoretical frameworks. Other mindfulness-based interventions are likely to have their own guidelines and recommendations for governance. (See Appendix 14.1 for a checklist of preparatory tasks for facilitators running mindfulness for psychosis groups.)

Prior Training as a Psychological or Mindfulness Practitioner

Mindfulness for psychosis is explicitly framed as a psychological therapy. Therefore, at least one facilitator needs to have completed a foundational training either as a psychological practitioner or therapist, or as a mindfulness practitioner (see Figure 14.1). Completing a recognized practitioner training ensures a solid foundation from which to develop further skills and knowledge in facilitating mindfulness for psychosis groups, and adherence to a professional code of conduct.

First let us consider the psychological practitioner or therapist pathway. This could be met by holding a relevant professional registration or license (e.g., as a clinical or counseling psychologist), or by being accredited by a nationally recognized professional body in a particular therapeutic modality (e.g., as a cognitive-behavioral therapist or dialectical behavior therapist).

Regarding a foundational training in mindfulness, we recommend a training pathway that confers readiness to offer mindfulness training developed for people with physical or mental health conditions, such as mindfulness-based stress reduction (MBSR; Kabat-Zinn, 2013) and mindfulness-based cognitive therapy (MBCT; Segal, Williams, et al.,

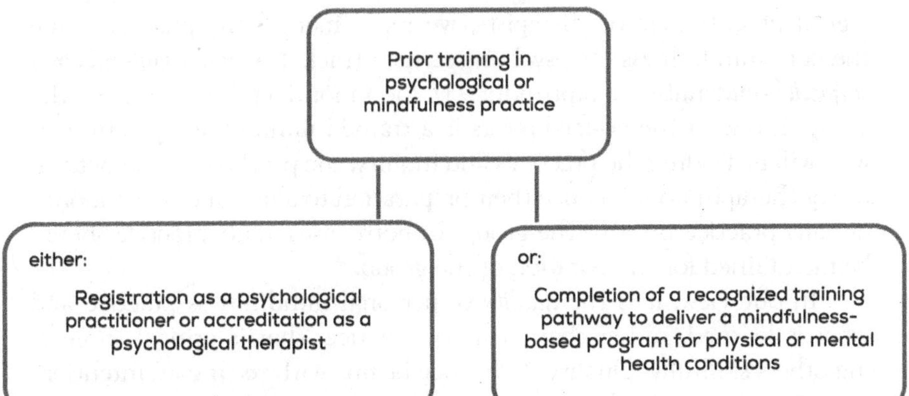

FIGURE 14.1. Foundational training requirements for facilitating mindfulness for psychosis groups.

2002). The mindfulness program in which people are trained should be based on an explicit psychological model of the relevant physical or mental health condition.

Prior training in facilitating groups is beneficial but not a prerequisite. This book aims to provide sufficient guidance for a trained psychological or mindfulness practitioner to understand and support the relevant therapeutic factors over the eight-session program. That said, seeking out opportunities for broader development as a group facilitator is helpful.

Establishing a Daily Mindfulness Practice

Mindfulness for psychosis group facilitators should themselves have an established daily practice. People trained to deliver evidence-based mindfulness programs, such as MBSR and MBCT, are likely to have an established personal practice. This probably involves practices that differ somewhat from the core mindfulness practice; we encourage prospective facilitators to incorporate the mindfulness for psychosis practice into their personal routine for at least 4 weeks prior to running the group, and maintaining this for the duration of the eight-session program.

Psychological practitioners and therapists are less likely to have an established personal practice. If the group is to be led by two psychological practitioners or therapists, we recommend daily practice using the core mindfulness for psychosis script (Track 1 at *www.guilford.com/chadwick-materials*; see Appendix 9.1), for 3 months prior to starting the group. If one of the co-facilitators is a trained mindfulness practitioner who will be leading the practices and inquiry, the psychological practitioner or therapist could reduce their preparation to a minimum of 1 month of daily practice prior to the group. In both cases, daily practice should be maintained for the duration of the group.

In our view, it is the *quality* of personal mindfulness practice and what is learned, rather than years of practice, that is critical to guiding others skillfully. Quality of practice begins with setting an intention, and we encourage facilitators to begin their daily mindfulness practice by connecting with an intention to support people with distressing psychosis using this approach. Facilitators vary in their knowledge and experience of mindfulness theory and practice, and should always be transparent about this with others, including their supervisor, co-facilitator, and group members. We recommend seeking guidance, mentoring, or supervision from an experienced mindfulness practitioner, where possible.

Mindfulness Practice Journal for Facilitators

The weekly mindfulness practice journal for facilitators is designed to support regular practice and reflective learning (see Figure 14.2 and Appendix 14.2). The journal prompts self-reflection and metacognitive insights that will inform peer discussion (with the co-facilitator) and supervision (see below), to enhance facilitation skills.

When completing the journal, we encourage facilitators to engage thoughtfully with each question, revisiting and sharpening emerging responses. Our experience is that facilitators who give time to this process and engage fully with each item work with the group more skillfully when this commences. The nature of journal reflections is likely to reflect the core process of change articulated in this book. As we deepen our practice and understanding, alongside discovery of helpful metacognitive insights, we will encounter unhelpful metacognitive beliefs and self-judgments, and these are opportunities for self-compassion and self-acceptance. Observing and learning from the process unfolding in ourselves enhances our facilitation of mindfulness for psychosis groups.

We recommend that new facilitators complete the mindfulness practice journal for at least 4 weeks prior to running the group (and that co-facilitators complete the journal separately) and then discuss this in weekly peer or supervisory meetings over the month preparing for the group, and for the full duration of the group. Facilitators may wish to add further rows for additional personally relevant prompts.

Cultivating Compassionate Self-Reflection of Beliefs That Threaten the Process of Change

The following scenario illustrates how we can become preoccupied with our own concerns in mindfulness for psychosis groups, and how we can prompt ourselves to let these go. We describe this from the perspectives of the facilitator, Lara, and the group members in Session 1.

Mindfulness practice **Date:** *Week 3*	**Reflections, learning, actions**
How was my practice last week?	*Practiced most mornings. Helped to feel calm and focused at the start of the day.*
What stands out from my practice?	*Sense of calm and how pleasant this feels. Some frustration that I spent so little time feeling like this.*
What have I learned about my mind and body?	*It's all so changeable. My mind jumps around all over the place and my body is sometimes really tense even when I don't notice this.*
What have I learned about being with difficult experiences?	*It's all about how I respond. Occasionally I can step back, and this feels empowering. More often, I've already reacted before I even notice.*
What have I learned about distress and suffering in my life?	*It's still there! I react to difficult memories quickly and get lost in these, going around and around in my mind and waste so much time.*
What have I observed about my habitual patterns of reactivity?	*There's a moment when I first react when I could step back but I almost choose to go with it. Stepping back then gets harder and harder.*
How has mindfulness influenced how I am in stressful situations?	*It feels empowering to step back and not react to the "heat" in my body. When I "lose it" and react it feels bad; I don't like who I become.*
How accepting have I been—of myself, others, my experiences?	*I had a setback and felt OK about it. I started to judge myself but then noticed what I was doing and let go of my usual way of reacting.*
What have I learned from ad hoc moments of mindfulness?	*I can tune back into my breath and body even in busy, difficult situations with lots of other people around—I feel more in control when I do this.*
What have I learned from moments of joy, connection?	*They are always there. I can choose to notice and be open to them. I feel more connected to other people and nature when I do this.*
Anything else from this week?	*My formal mindfulness practice has slipped over the last few days, and I've noticed the impact. I'll practice each morning again next week.*

FIGURE 14.2. Weekly mindfulness practice journal for facilitators—illustrative example.

Lara's Perspective

Lara has been planning the mindfulness for psychosis group for over 3 months. This is the first group she is leading, and it was not possible to find a co-facilitator. Leading up to the program starting, she felt excited—she is committed to working with people with psychosis, and mindfulness sits well with her values. She also felt familiar fleeting anxieties and doubts: "*What if only one or two people show up, or there are lots of dropouts, or people just don't benefit?*"

It's now over halfway through Session 1. Seven people came, which is great! Lara is leading inquiry after the second practice. The anxiety in the room is still high. Lara can't tell how well mindfulness is landing or how much people are connecting with her or other group members; people seem quieter and less talkative than at the start.

Lara begins to worry she is *losing the group* and imagines colleagues talking if the group goes badly or folds. She would like to feel more at ease but can't right now. She is feeling slightly cut off from the group. She notices some people seem distracted and worries they are thinking this isn't really what they need and may not benefit. She feels under pressure and a little stressed. Lara has an urge to revisit the psychoeducation and push the key points more, to really explain how mindfulness could help. She wishes she had a co-facilitator to share the responsibility.

At this point, Lara remembers her supervisor saying: "*As best you can, trust mindfulness and trust the group members.*" This helps her reset, and for a few moments she settles back into her breathing and body. She once again feels connected to the people who made it to the session today—not an easy thing for them to have done. She smiles and asks an open question, happy to leave ample space for people to contribute, interested to hear what people will say next.

Group Members' Perspectives

Halfway through Session 1, most of the group members are feeling tired, many having slept badly the night before this initial meeting. Several were kept awake by voices, paranoia, and worry about the new group: "*What if I can't do the mindfulness?; What if I don't fit in with the others?*" It might be too much. Some people's voices warned them that the group was dangerous. One person's voices told him they were going to experiment on him. For all seven people who made it here, traveling to the session was quite stressful.

The group members had found Session 1 OK so far. Nothing big had happened, which was reassuring. When Lara had said two people were missing, everyone who was there could understand why. They all appreciated Lara thanking them for being there and saying how normal it is to feel anxious about joining a group and meeting new people.

Most people found the mindfulness practice OK. Some were worried that 10 minutes sounded like a long time, though this had passed more quickly than expected. Everyone found it difficult to stay focused and present during the practice—Lara's guidance helped them refocus when their mind had wandered. The main thing people understood was that mindfulness meant taking some time to just stop—*stepping back* as Lara called it—and notice their breathing and what was going on in their body and mind. Most were encouraged when Lara had said noticing your mind wandering was the starting point of mindfulness and everyone had done some of this.

It was a relief that there weren't too many questions, and that there didn't seem to be right or wrong answers. Nobody was shot down for saying the wrong thing. Lara's responses made each person feel a little safer—like they'd said something important (though she didn't go over the top). There were some uncomfortable silences when Lara asked something about mindfulness and no one replied. It was hard to think with the intrusive voices, images, and thoughts during both the practice and discussions. Some people talked about their voices and fears, others talked about difficult thoughts and images, and everyone noticed how they had something in common with at least one other person in the group.

Two people were getting a lot of self-critical thoughts and voices, telling them they were talking rubbish, and no longer felt able to say anything. They were glad that Lara let them just listen and didn't put them on the spot. By now, most had begun worrying about traveling home. Children would be getting out of school, and this made the voices and paranoia worse for some people. They were all glad they would be getting a handout as it would be hard to remember much once they got home.

Responding Mindfully to Facilitator Beliefs That Threaten the Process of Change

In mindfulness for psychosis groups, we are cultivating kind, compassionate self-reflection in order to foster people's ability to respond mindfully to difficult internal experience. This applies to facilitators as well as group members.

Facilitators often have moments of anxiety and doubt both leading up to and during sessions. As illustrated by Lara's concerns, facilitators commonly worry that the group will *go badly*, that people won't *get it*, and so will drop out or not benefit. These fears can be triggered in sessions by people appearing not to engage, fewer people attending than expected, someone deciding not to return, or specific comments, for example, a group member saying: "*This group has just got to work; I can't keep going on like this.*" There may also be linked concerns about what our colleagues will think if the group doesn't go well.

Many of these concerns are surface expressions of facilitators' underlying beliefs about not being good enough, not being up to the task, feelings about failing group members, or similar self-evaluative judgments. Having spent many years involved in training psychologists and psychological therapists, we know how critically some judge themselves. Beliefs and assumptions about personal responsibility and the nature of psychosis are similarly problematic. Facilitators can feel responsible for group members engaging and benefiting from the group, and at the same time feeling somehow different and distant from people with psychosis (see Table 14.1).

Unexamined and unchecked, implicit beliefs about ourselves, psychosis, and personal responsibility can *threaten the process of change.* These beliefs leak into awareness in the form of streams of thoughts and

TABLE 14.1. Disempowering Facilitator Beliefs

Beliefs about responsibility for engagement and change	Beliefs about psychosis
I'm responsible for keeping people in the group.	People with psychosis are dangerous, unpredictable, and I'll say the wrong thing and upset them.
I'm responsible for people improving.	I (alone) must keep them safe.
I'm responsible for preventing aggression and harm.	We won't connect as people because of the things they hear, see, and believe (hallucinations, delusions).
Getting people to change shows colleagues and the wider service my worth.	People with psychosis are too vulnerable and ill to learn mindfulness or make decisions for themselves.

fleeting images. In the situation above, Lara starts to focus on anxieties about what the group members are thinking, how mindfulness is landing with them, whether they are connecting with her or one another, what her colleagues might think, and whether she should have delayed the group until a co-facilitator could join her.

These streams of thoughts and images distract facilitators, pulling their attention toward their own internal dialogue and away from members of the group. This conflicts with the need to attend to the unfolding events in the session, and obscures the attitudinal qualities of authenticity, acceptance, and trust, that support the therapeutic group factors, thereby threatening the core process of change. Furthermore, when facilitators are caught in the grip of self-judgment and doubt, they too suffer.

We are all susceptible to such anxieties and doubts. When these inevitably arise, we seek to recognize them and, as best we can, allow them to pass or fade. We bring these momentary anxieties and doubts to peer reflection or supervision, holding them with self-compassion and as learning opportunities.

In summary, in group sessions, we seek to (1) recognize and step back from fears and beliefs as they arise; (2) lean back into the qualities of authenticity, acceptance, and trust; and (3) tune back into the experience of members of the group, to support the group factors and core process of change. Lara was able to recall her supervisor's advice to "*trust mindfulness and trust the group members.*" This helped her take a few moments to focus on her own breathing, and then turn her attention back to the group and facilitate the discussion, calmly and effectively.

Postgroup reflection and supervision are opportunities to increase awareness and moment-to-moment recognition of our own habitual fears, worries, judgments, and reactions, and to hold these with self-compassion and a sense of universality. This can be done by focusing on moments of anxiety, despondency, and other emotions that arose when facilitating the group, and exploring independently or in supervision: "*Where did I feel this in my body?*" "*What thoughts, images, and memories came to mind, or come to mind when focusing on this feeling?*" "*Do any responsibility beliefs arise?*" "*Any unspoken beliefs about psychosis?*" "*Any other assumptions or beliefs about myself, mindfulness, or people with psychosis?*" Articulating and cultivating alternative *empowering* beliefs can also enable us to let go of our unhelpful beliefs (see Table 14.2).

TABLE 14.2. Alternative, Empowering Facilitator Beliefs

Empowering attitude to engagement and change in mindfulness for psychosis groups	Empowering beliefs about psychosis
My responsibility is do my best, moment-to-moment, offering the program in an ethical, mindful, and trusting way, and accepting each person's right to determine their own path to recovery.	• Psychosis is not the person—people are so much more than their psychosis. • My responsibility regarding risk is to act ethically and professionally, and do my best. • In a therapeutic setting that is accepting and empowering, people with psychosis find their own paths to recovery.

A Mindful Approach Immediately Prior to Group Sessions

Immediately prior to group sessions, take a few moments to tune in to your body, mind, and emotions. Is there any worry, fear, stress, reactivity? If so, take a moment to ask, "*What beliefs are lying behind this feeling?*" Can you label these (e.g., "*I'm assuming too much responsibility*" or "*I'm not trusting the group*")? Perhaps ask yourself, "*What is lacking in this moment?*" (e.g., acceptance, letting go). Look out for worries about not getting through all the material or an urge to be overly goal driven (e.g., "*Let's get this done*"). Step back and consider alternatives that allow you to respond with curiosity (e.g., "*I wonder who'll surprise me today in the group*"). As best you can, return to the facilitator qualities of authenticity, acceptance, and trust. Remind yourself that we are all prone to these anxieties and doubts from time to time, including us, the authors of this book.

Coming Back to a Mindful Approach during Group Sessions

During sessions, give yourself time. Breathe and observe your inner experience. If you feel stress, anxiety, or other emotions arise, take a moment to pause, step back, and breathe before speaking. As best you can, maintain an awareness of your emotional, mental, and physical state, to guide you. Accept whatever is present with kindness and compassion—there is no need to judge yourself.

If you are feeling anxious or worried, as best you can, allow these feelings to be fully present. This brings self-compassion and acceptance. Occasionally, we might share that we were having a moment of doubt or mild worry—this normalizes and embodies acceptance of these feelings. Remind yourself that these anxieties and concerns seem to be universal among the caring professions. If it helps, try silently noting what is present and opening out awareness. Come back to the attitudinal qualities of authenticity, acceptance, and trust. You are doing your best.

Postgroup Self-Reflection and Supervision

Always plan on at least 15 minutes after sessions for either peer reflection or supervision (we recognize that finding and funding expert supervision is not always possible). Postgroup reflection is less about checking content ("*Yes, we did that*") and more about reflecting on the process and embodiment of mindful acceptance ("*How was that?*"). The *postsession reflection scale* is designed to guide peer discussion and supervision (see Figure 14.3 and Appendix 14.3). Facilitators can complete this separately or together and then discuss.

End-of-Group Reflection and Learning

At the end of an eight-session mindfulness for psychosis program, it is important to review and reflect on the program as a whole in order to learn and develop as facilitators. We recommend reviewing all completed postsession reflection scales as part of this review. This process may identify further training and professional development needs. It can also be helpful to present a summary of the group to colleagues or students, and seek feedback from people familiar and unfamiliar with the details of the group. Try not to become preoccupied with perfection—this tends to stifle learning for both facilitators and group members. As best you can, come back to the qualities of authenticity, acceptance, and trust, and enjoy the groups and learning from people with psychosis how best to live well with these experiences.

Date: *December 1, 2025* **Session:** *3* **Core facilitator skills**	**Score (1–5)**	**When did this go well today?**	**When did this go less well today?**	**Reflections, learning, actions**
1. Active listening and validation	*4*	*In psychoeducation—more people talked after this*	*When X spoke at some length—needed to move on*	*Take to supervision*
2. Embodying authenticity, acceptance, and trust	*3–4*	*In inquiry—felt attuned to people's emotions*	*Started to feel frustrated when X was speaking*	*I can get frustrated when feeling overresponsible and worried about not doing things well enough*
3. Summarizing and reflecting	*4*	*In inquiry—also linking people's experiences*	*Some opportunities missed*	*Listen for opportunities to use summaries, accept that we can't pick up everything*
4. Ensuring structure and pacing aligns with people's needs	*3*	*OK through most of the session*	*A bit rushed at the end*	*Make sure we get to the break by the halfway point on the agenda*
5. Supporting universality, cohesion, hope, being oneself more fully	*3*	*Made links between S and K's experiences*	*Could have drawn out other links and conveyed hope more*	*As for summaries above—link people's experiences; highlight expressions of hope*
6. Supporting understanding of metacognitive beliefs and insights	*2–3*	*Started to draw out "reacting creates suffering"*	*Missed opportunity to link this to choice (focus of session)*	*Listen for metacognitive beliefs/insights and highlight these when they arise*
7. Attending to the overall aim for the session	*3*	*Introduced "choice" and wove into guided practice*	*As above and could have made more links in inquiry*	*Draw out session theme more clearly and link to comments in inquiry and psychoeducation*
8. Being present during the session today	*3–4*	*Fair for first half of session*	*Less present when X started talking a lot*	*Take to supervision—discuss how to manage my reactions when unsettled*
What have you learned from today's session—what stands out given these reflections?	*Session went well in terms of validating people's experiences. Some people contributed who hadn't spoken before. Was thrown when X started talking a lot—take to supervision to discuss best response for all.*			

FIGURE 14.3. Mindfulness for psychosis groups—example of facilitator postsession reflection scale.

A Community of Mindfulness for Psychosis Facilitators

Our intention in writing this book is to offer clear guidance on facilitating mindfulness for psychosis groups, and to support the development of a community of learners. Having read the full text, we hope you now have all you need to start facilitating these groups. We strongly encourage you to use the chapters and session guidance as a resource and return to relevant sections repeatedly to clarify and deepen your theoretical understanding and improve your clinical practice.

As humans we are intrinsically social learners. Writing this book was only possible through many, many conversations among us to clarify the principles, theory, and practice outlined here. Connecting with a community of practitioners and researchers will deepen your experiential understanding of mindfulness, and how to introduce this in a way that is accessible and therapeutic for people with psychosis. Our hope is that in addition to using this book to facilitate groups, you will now reach out to others who are also seeking to become skillful mindfulness facilitators. In this way, we can collectively support people living with the tyranny of psychosis to empower themselves through mindfulness, find greater self-acceptance, and in doing so regain a sense of common humanity and recover the lives they choose to lead.

APPENDIX 14.1. Mindfulness for Psychosis Groups—Preparatory Tasks for New Facilitators

Preparatory tasks	Check
1. Read this book and discuss questions and reflections regularly (over a period of at least 1 month) in supervision.	
2. Establish a daily practice incorporating the core mindfulness for psychosis guidance (at least 3 months if neither co-facilitator is mindfulness trained; otherwise 1 month).	
3. Keep a weekly mindfulness practice journal, and bring reflections to supervision.	
4. Identify a co-facilitator who can fully commit to preparing for and running a mindfulness for psychosis group.	
5. Ensure at least one facilitator has therapeutic experience working with people with psychosis.	
6. Organize weekly supervision for the month prior to starting the group, and the full duration of the group.	
7. Logistics: Make referrers aware; agree on referral and assessment processes; identify and book room; collate materials including recordings.	
8. Be able to describe the two-circles model, simply and succinctly.	
9. Be able to describe the core process of change, simply and succinctly.	
10. Be able to guide the core mindfulness practice and outline the three *moments of mindfulness*.	
11. Agree with co-facilitator and supervisor how you will use the Facilitator Postsession Reflection Scale.	
12. Immediately prior to group sessions: Take a few moments to tune in to your body, mind, and emotions.	

APPENDIX 14.2. Mindfulness for Psychosis Groups— Facilitator Weekly Practice Journal

Note. This can be a helpful way to monitor your development as a mindfulness facilitator.

Mindfulness practice **Date: ___________**	**Reflections, learning, actions**
How was my practice last week?	
What stands out from my practice?	
What have I learned about my mind and body?	
What have I learned about being with difficult experiences?	
What have I learned about distress and suffering in my life?	
What have I observed about my habitual patterns of reactivity?	
How has mindfulness influenced how I am in stressful situations?	
How accepting have I been of myself, others, my experiences?	
What have I learned from ad hoc moments of mindfulness?	
What have I learned from moments of joy, connection?	
Anything else from this week?	

From *Mindfulness for Psychosis: A Group Therapy Approach*, by Paul Chadwick, Katherine Newman-Taylor, and Nicola Abba. Copyright © 2027 The Guilford Press. Permission to photocopy this material, or to download and print enlarged versions (*www.guilford.com/chadwick-materials*), is granted to purchasers of this book for personal use or use with clients; see copyright page for details.

APPENDIX 14.3. Mindfulness for Psychosis Groups—Facilitator Postsession Reflection Scale

Note. This tool can help you evaluate your fluency with various components of the therapy.

Date: ________ **Session:** ________ **Core facilitator skills**	**Score (1–5)**	**When did this go well today?**	**When did this go less well today?**	**Reflections, learning, actions**
1. Active listening and validation				
2. Embodying authenticity, acceptance, and trust				
3. Summarizing and reflecting				
4. Ensuring structure and pacing aligns with people's needs				
5. Supporting universality, cohesion, hope, being oneself more fully				
6. Supporting understanding of metacognitive beliefs and insights				
7. Attending to the overall aim for the session				
8. Being present during the session today				
What have you learned from today's session: What stands out given these reflections?				

From *Mindfulness for Psychosis: A Group Therapy Approach*, by Paul Chadwick, Katherine Newman-Taylor, and Nicola Abba. Copyright © 2027 The Guilford Press. Permission to photocopy this material, or to download and print enlarged versions (*www.guilford.com/chadwick-materials*), is granted to purchasers of this book for personal use or use with clients; see copyright page for details.

References

Abba, N., Chadwick, P., & Stevenson, C. (2008). Responding mindfully to distressing psychosis: A grounded theory analysis. *Psychotherapy Research, 18*(1), 77–87.

Austin, S. F., Mors, O., Budtz-Jørgensen, E., Secher, R. G., Hjorthøj, C. R., Bertelsen, M., et al. (2015). Long-term trajectories of positive and negative symptoms in first episode psychosis: A 10-year follow-up study in the opus cohort. *Schizophrenia Research, 168*(1–2), 84–91.

Beck, A. T. (1979). *Cognitive therapy and the emotional disorders*. Penguin.

Chadwick, P. (2006). *Person-based cognitive therapy for distressing psychosis*. Wiley.

Chadwick, P. (2019). Mindfulness for psychosis: Humanising therapeutic process. *Current Opinion in Psychology, 28*, 317–320.

Chadwick, P., & Birchwood, M. (1994). The omnipotence of voices: A cognitive approach to auditory hallucinations. *British Journal of Psychiatry, 164*(2), 190–201.

Chadwick, P., Birchwood, M. J., & Trower, P. (1996). *Cognitive therapy for delusions, voices and paranoia*. Wiley.

Chadwick, P., Hughes, S., Russell, D., Russell, I., & Dagnan, D. (2009). Mindfulness groups for distressing voices and paranoia: A replication and randomized feasibility trial. *Behavioural and Cognitive Psychotherapy, 37*(4), 403–412.

Chadwick, P., Newman-Taylor, K., & Abba, N. (2005). Mindfulness groups for people with psychosis. *Behavioural and Cognitive Psychotherapy, 33*(3), 351–359.

Ellett, L. (2024). Mindfulness for psychosis: Current evidence, unanswered questions and future directions. *Psychology and Psychotherapy: Theory, Research and Practice, 97*(1), 34–40.

Garety, P. A., Kuipers, E., Fowler, D., Freeman, D., & Bebbington, P. E. (2001). A cognitive model of the positive symptoms of psychosis. *Psychological Medicine, 31*(2), 189–195.

Glaser, B., & Strauss, A. (1967). *The discovery of grounded theory: Strategies for qualitative research*. Aldine de Gruyter.

Gumley, A., Schwannauer, M., MacBeth, A., & Read, J. (2008). Emotional recovery and staying well after psychosis: An attachment-based conceptualisation. *Attachment: New Directions in Psychotherapy and Relational Psychoanalysis, 2*(2), 127–148.

Hayes, L. J. (1994). Thinking. In S. C. Hayes, L. J. Hayes, M. Sato, & K. Ono (Eds.), *Behavior analysis of language and cognition* (pp. 149–164). Context Press/New Harbinger.

Hayes, S. C. (2002). Acceptance, mindfulness, and science. *Clinical Psychology: Science and Practice, 9*(1), 101–106.

Hodann-Caudevilla, R. M., Díaz-Silveira, C., Burgos-Julián, F. A., & Santed, M. A. (2020). Mindfulness-based interventions for people with schizophrenia: A systematic review and meta-analysis. *International Journal of Environmental Research and Public Health, 17*(13), 4690.

Humphrey, N. (1993). *A history of the mind*. Vintage

Jansen, J. E., Gleeson, J., Bendall, S., Rice, S., & Alvarez-Jimenez, M. (2020). Acceptance- and mindfulness-based interventions for persons with psychosis: A systematic review and meta-analysis. *Schizophrenia Research, 215*, 25–37.

Jaspers, K. (1913/1997). *General psychopathology* (J. Hoenig & M. W. Hamilton, Trans.; 7th ed.). Johns Hopkins University Press. (Original work published 1913)

Kabat-Zinn, J. (1990). *Full catastrophe living: How to cope with stress, pain and illness using mindfulness meditation*. Hachette UK.

Kabat-Zinn, J. (1994). *Wherever you go, there you are: Mindfulness meditation in everyday life*. Hyperion.

Kabat-Zinn, J. (2013). *Full catastrophe living: How to cope with stress, pain and illness using mindfulness meditation* (rev. ed.). Hachette UK.

Kahneman, D. (2011). *Fast and slow thinking*. Allen Lane & Penguin Books.

Kingdon, D. G., & Turkington, D. (2022). *Cognitive-behavioral therapy of schizophrenia*. Psychology Press.

Lacan, J. (1993). *The psychoses*. WW Norton & Company.

Larkin, A., & Hutton, P. (2017). Systematic review and meta-analysis of factors that help or hinder treatment decision-making capacity in psychosis. *British Journal of Psychiatry, 211*(4), 205–215.

Liu, B., Zhao, H., & Lu, Q. (2021). Effect of leader mindfulness on hindrance stress in nurses: The social mindfulness information processing path. *Journal of Advanced Nursing, 77*(11), 4414–4426.

McCarthy-Jones, S., Barnes, L. J., Hill, G. E., Marwood, L., Moseley, P., & Fernyhough, C. (2011). When words and pictures come alive: Relating the modality of intrusive thoughts to modalities of hypnagogic/hypnopompic hallucinations. *Personality and Individual Differences, 51*(6), 787–790.

McGlanaghy, E., Turner, D., Davis, G. A., Sharpe, H., Dougall, N., Morris, P., et al.

(2021). A network meta-analysis of psychological interventions for schizophrenia and psychosis: Impact on symptoms. *Schizophrenia Research, 228*, 447–459.

Morrison, A. P. (2001). The interpretation of intrusions in psychosis: An integrative cognitive approach to hallucinations and delusions. *Behavioural and Cognitive Psychotherapy, 29*(3), 257–276.

Nelson, H. E. (2005). *Cognitive-behavioural therapy with delusions and hallucinations: A practice manual.* Thornes.

Newman-Taylor, K., & Abba, N. (2013). Mindfulness mit psychose. In A. Knuf & M. Hammer (Eds.), *Die Entdeckung der Achtsamkeit in der Arbeit mit Psychisch Erkrankten Menschen* (pp. 134–150). Psychiatrie Verlag.

Newman-Taylor, K., & Abba, N. (2015). Mindfulness meditation in CBT for psychosis. In B. A. Gaudiano (Ed.), *Incorporating acceptance and mindfulness into the treatment of psychosis: Current trends and future directions* (pp. 170–200). Oxford University Press.

Newman-Taylor, K., & Abba, N. (2018). Mindfulness in CBT for psychosis. In C. Cupitt (Ed.), *CBT for psychosis* (pp. 64–78). Routledge.

Newman-Taylor, K., Graves, A., & Stopa, L. (2008). Strategic cognition in paranoia: The use of thought control strategies in a non-clinical population. *Behavioural and Cognitive Psychotherapy, 37*(1), 25–38.

Newman Taylor, K., Harper, S., & Chadwick, P. (2009). Impact of mindfulness on cognition and affect in voice hearing: Evidence from two case studies. *Behavioural and Cognitive Psychotherapy, 37*(4), 397–402.

O'Brien-Venus, B., Jenkins, T., & Chadwick, P. (2023). Self-dehumanisation in voice hearers: The end of a continuum. *Frontiers in Psychiatry, 14*, 1173380.

O'Brien-Venus, B., Ellett, L., Burgess-Barr, S., & Chadwick, P. (2024). Systematic review of the safety of mindfulness-based interventions for psychosis. *Clinical Psychology Review, 112*, 102445.

O'Donoghue, E. K., Morris, E. M., Oliver, J., & Johns, L. C. (2018). *ACT for psychosis recovery: A practical manual for group-based interventions using acceptance and commitment therapy.* New Harbinger.

Padesky, C. A. (1993, September 24). *Socratic questioning: Changing minds or guiding discovery.* Paper presented at the European Congress of Behavioural and Cognitive Therapies, London.

Padesky, C. A., & Kennerley, H. (2023). *Dialogues for discovery: Improving psychotherapy's effectiveness.* Oxford University Press.

Proctor, K., Wood, R., & Newman-Taylor, K. (2019). Welcoming peer workers in NHS settings: Facilitating readiness with an early intervention in psychosis team. *Mental Health and Social Inclusion, 23*(1), 30–35.

Rahula, W. (1959). *What the Buddha taught.* Oneworld Publications.

Rogers, C. R. (1961). *On becoming a person: A therapist's view of psychotherapy.* Constable.

Rogers, C. R., & Farson, R. E. (1957). *Active listening.* University of Chicago.

Romme, M. A., Honig, A., Noorthoorn, E. O., & Escher, A. D. (1992). Coping

with hearing voices: An emancipatory approach. *British Journal of Psychiatry, 161*(1), 99–103.
Romme, M. A. J., & Escher, A. D. M. A. C. (1989). Hearing voices. *Schizophrenia Bulletin, 15*(2), 209–216.
Safran, J., & Segal, Z. V. (1996). *Interpersonal process in cognitive therapy*. Aronson.
Segal, Z. V., Teasdale, J. D., Williams, J. M., & Gemar, M. C. (2002). The Mindfulness-Based Cognitive Therapy Adherence Scale: Inter-rater reliability, adherence to protocol and treatment distinctiveness. *Clinical Psychology and Psychotherapy, 9*(2), 131–138.
Segal, Z. V., Williams, J. M. G., & Teasdale, J. D. (2002). *Mindfulness-based cognitive therapy for depression: A new approach to preventing relapse*. Guilford Press.
Sellers, R., Varese, F., Wells, A., & Morrison, A. P. (2017). A meta-analysis of metacognitive beliefs as implicated in the self-regulatory executive function model in clinical psychosis. *Schizophrenia Research, 179*, 75–84.
Skrobinska, L., Newman-Taylor, K., & Carnelley, K. (2024). Psychosis and help-seeking behaviour—A systematic review of the literature. *Psychology and Psychotherapy: Theory, Research and Practice, 97*(4), 583–605.
Teasdale, J. D. (1993). Emotion and two kinds of meaning: Cognitive therapy and applied cognitive science. *Behaviour Research and Therapy, 31*, 339–354.
Teasdale, J. D., Moore, R. G., Hayhurst, H., Pope, M., Williams, S., & Segal, Z. V. (2002). Metacognitive awareness and prevention of relapse in depression: Empirical evidence. *Journal of Consulting and Clinical Psychology, 70*(2), 275–287.
Teasdale, J. D., Segal, Z. V., & Williams, J. M. (2003). Mindfulness training and problem formulation. *Clinical Psychology: Science and Practice, 10*(2), 157–160.
Williams, J. M. (2008). Mindfulness, depression and modes of mind. *Cognitive Therapy and Research, 32*(6), 721–733.
Williams, J. M. (2010). Mindfulness and psychological process. *Emotion, 10*(1), 1–7.
Woods, A. (2011). *The sublime object of psychiatry: Schizophrenia in clinical and cultural theory*. OUP.
Yalom, I. D. (1995). *The theory and practice of group psychotherapy*. Basic Books.

Index

Note. t or *f* following a page number indicates a table or a figure.

B

C

D

H

I

R

S

U

V

W